ELECTROCARDIOGRAPHY
FOR HEALTH CARE PERSONNEL

Second Edition

Kathryn A. Booth, RN-BSN, MS, RMA

Total Care Programming
Palm Coast, Florida

Patricia DeiTos, RN, MSN

Inova Health System
Fairfax, Virginia

Thomas E. O'Brien, MBA, BBA, AS, CCT

Central Florida Institute
Palm Harbor, Florida

 Higher Education

Boston   Burr Ridge, IL   Dubuque, IA   New York   San Francisco   St. Louis
Bangkok   Bogotá   Caracas   Kuala Lumpur   Lisbon   London   Madrid   Mexico City
Milan   Montreal   New Delhi   Santiago   Seoul   Singapore   Sydney   Taipei   Toronto

The McGraw·Hill Companies

Higher Education

ELECTROCARDIOGRAPHY FOR HEALTH CARE PERSONNEL, SECOND EDITION

ISBN 978–0–07–351098–9
MHID 0–07–351098–X

Editor-in-Chief: *Elizabeth J. Haefele*
Senior Sponsoring Editor: *Roxan Kinsey*
Developmental Editor: *Connie Kuhl*
Senior Marketing Manager: *Nancy Bradshaw*
Senior Project Manager: *Sheila M. Frank*
Senior Production Supervisor: *Sherry L. Kane*
Media Producer: *Benjamin Curless*
Media Project Manager: *Mark A. S. Dierker*
Designer: *Laurie B. Janssen*
Cover Designer: *Studio Montage*
(USE) Cover Image: *Photodisc: Medicine Today, V59*
Senior Photo Research Coordinator: *Lori Hancock*
Photo Research: *LouAnn K. Wilson*
Compositor: *Precision Graphics*
Typeface: *11/13 Melior*
Printer: *Quebecor World Versailles, KY*

The credits section for this book begins on page 285 and is considered an extension of the copyright page.

Library of Congress Cataloging-in-Publication Data

Booth, Kathryn A., 1957-
    Electrocardiology for health care personnel / Kathryn A. Booth, Patricia DeiTos,
    Thomas O'Brien. – 2nd ed.
        p. cm.
    Rev. ed. of: Glencoe electrocardiography for health care personnel / Kathryn A. Booth.
    ISBN 978–0–07–351098–9 — ISBN 0–07–351098–X
    1.   Electrocardiography. I. DeiTos, Patricia, 1957- II. O'Brien, Thomas (Thomas E.)
    III. Booth, Kathryn A., 1957- Glencoe electrocardiography for health care personnel. IV. Title.

RC683.5.E5H256 2008
616.1'207547–dc22

2007061184

www.mhhe.com

Dedication

To the students who are using this book. Thank you for choosing the field of health care for your career. Your skills and services are truly needed. To my daughter Carrie who helps me gets things done.

Kathyrn Booth

I would like to dedicate this book to my husband Dick and my lovely children Kristin, Pete, and Melissa who provided the support and encouragement to pursue my goals and dreams.

Patricia DeiTos

I want to thank my beautiful wife Michele and our wonderful children Thomas, Robert, and Kathryn. Without their love and support, I would have nothing. They inspire me every day to make a difference in people's lives. I also want to express my sincere thanks to the faculty, staff, and students of Central Florida Institute for their encouragement and guidance. Today's students are the difference makers of tomorrow!

Thomas O'Brien

About the Authors

Kathryn A. Booth, RN, BSN, MS, RMA, is a full-time author, educator, and consultant for Total Care Programming, a multimedia software development company. Her background includes a bachelor's degree in nursing and a master's degree in education. Her 27 years of teaching, nursing, and health care work experience span four states. She has authored and developed multimedia software and health care textbooks and educational materials for McGraw-Hill Higher Education; Total Care Programming; Glencoe/McGraw-Hill; Mosby Lifeline; and Lippincott, Williams, and Wilkins. Kathy Booth has presented at numerous state, corporate, and national conventions since 1994. Her current focus is to develop up-to-date, dynamic health care education materials to assist educators and promote the health care profession. To remain current, Kathy has most recently worked as a part-time LPN instructor and a practicing medical assistant, and she has just completed her RMA certification.

Patricia DeiTos, RN, MSN, WPD, is a full-time educator for Inova Health System, a large, nonprofit six-hospital system. Her background includes a bachelor's degree in nursing from Rush University and a master's degree in nursing administration from DePaul University. She received her certification in Professional in Workforce Development from the University of Virginia. Her experience includes over 27 years of diversified professional nursing, nursing education, and nursing management experience with specific focus on training, educational development, supervision, evaluation, and analysis of nursing staff and students. She has held positions in the following areas: first-line and middle-level management, critical care units, hospital, college, and private-sector-based education. Patti has presented at numerous state, local, and national conventions since 1995. Her current focus is on providing quality and appropriate education to the entry-level and beginning health care professional.

Thomas E. O'Brien, MBA, BBA, AS, CCT, MSgt USAF ret., is a full-time educator and Program Coordinator of Cardiovascular Technology at Central Florida Institute. He is also a subject matter consultant and test writer working with Cardiovascular Credentialing International (CCI) for the Certified Cardiographic Technician Registry Examination. His background includes over 24 years in the U.S. Air Force and U.S. Army Medical Corps. Tom O'Brien's medical career as an Air Force Independent Duty Medical Technician (IDMT) has taken him all over the United States and the world. Tom has several years experience working in the Emergency Services and Critical Care arena. He was awarded "Master Instructor" status by the U.S. Air Force in 1994 upon completion of his teaching practicum. He now has over 10 years of teaching experience; subjects include Emergency Medicine, Cardiovascular Nursing, Fundamentals of Nursing, Dysrhythmia, and 12-Lead ECG Interpretation. Tom is actively involved in book proposals, and he reviews for a number of publishers, including Glencoe/McGraw-Hill and Lippincott, Williams, and Wilkins. His current position provides challenges with the day-to-day development of curriculum to meet the ever-changing needs of the medical community and to provide first-rate education to a diverse adult education population.

Brief Contents

Contents

CHAPTER **7** Ambulatory Monitoring   206

Preface

Health care is an ever-changing and growing field. Flexibility is key to obtaining, maintaining, and improving your career. The concept of cross-training, or multiskilling, although not a new one, has become the expected rather than the exception. Cross-training allows you to be able to function in a variety of workplace settings doing diverse tasks. The fact that you are currently reading this book means that you are willing to acquire new skills or specialize the skills you already possess. This willingness translates into your enhanced value, job security, marketability, and mobility.

This second edition of *Electrocardiography for Health Care Personnel* was designed not just for classroom but also for independent and distance learning. Checkpoint Questions and student CD exercises have been added to make the learning process interactive and to promote increased comprehension. The variety of materials included with the program provides for multiple learning styles and ensures that you will be a success.

The text/workbook/CD is divided into seven chapters.

- *Chapter 1 Role of Electrocardiographer* introduces you into the field of electrocardiography and helps to promote the various roles in the field. You will also learn about the history and how ECGs are used.

- *Chapter 2 The Cardiovascular System* provides a complete introduction and review of the heart and its electrical system. The information focuses on what you "need to know" to understand and perform an ECG. Specific topics include anatomy of the heart, principles of circulation, cardiac cycle, conduction system and electrical stimulation, and the ECG waveform.

- *Chapter 3 The Electrocardiograph* creates a basic understanding of the ECG including producing the ECG waveform, the ECG machine, electrodes, and the ECG graph paper.

- *Chapter 4 Performing an ECG* describes the procedure for performing an ECG in a simple step-by-step fashion. Each part of the procedure is explained in detail taking into consideration the latest guidelines. The chapter is divided into the following topics: preparation, communication, anatomical landmarks, applying the electrodes and leads, safety and infection control, operating the ECG machine, checking the tracing, reporting results, and equipment maintenance. Extra sections are included regarding pediatric ECG, special patient circumstances, and emergencies. A competency checklist found in Appendix A provides the step-by-step procedure.

- *Chapter 5 ECG Interpretation and Clinical Significance* includes an introduction to dysrhythmias and all the basic dysrhythmias. Additional rhythms, ECG rhythm strips, figures, and exercises have been added to make this chapter easy to follow and comprehend.

- *Chapter 6 Exercise Electrocardiography* provides the information necessary to assist with an exercise electrocardiography. The competency checklist found in Appendix A will provide the step-by-step procedure for the student to become proficient at the skill.
- *Chapter 7 Ambulatory Monitoring* includes the latest information about various types of ambulatory monitors and includes what you need to know to apply and remove a monitor. A competency checklist is also provided in Appendix A for this skill.

Features of the Text/Workbook/CD

- **Key Terms, Glossary, and Audio Glossary:** Key terms are identified at the beginning of each chapter. These terms are in **bold** type within the chapter and are defined both in the chapter and in the glossary at the end of the book. Open the student CD to hear the pronunciation of each key term, and practice learning the term with the Key Term Concentration game.
- **Checkpoint Questions:** At the end of each main heading in the chapter are short-answer Checkpoint Questions. Answer these questions to make sure you have learned the basic concepts presented.
- **CD activities:** After you have finished the Checkpoint Questions, you are sent to the interactive student CD activity to further your review and practice of the concepts presented in each section. Be sure to complete the activities on the CD before you continue to the next section.
- **Troubleshooting:** The Troubleshooting feature identifies problems and situations that may arise when you are caring for patients or performing a procedure. At the end of this feature, you are asked a question to answer in your own words.
- **Safety and Infection Control:** You are responsible for providing safe care and preventing the spread of infection. This feature presents tips and techniques to help you practice these important skills relative to electrocardiography.
- **Patient Education and Communication:** Patient interaction and education and intrateam communication are integral parts of health care. As part of your daily duties, you must communicate effectively both orally and in writing, and you must provide patient education. Use this feature to learn ways to perform these tasks.
- **HIPAA, Law, and Ethics:** When working in health care, you must be conscious of the regulations of HIPAA (Health Insurance Portability and Accountability Act) and understand your legal responsibilities and the implications of your actions. You must perform duties within established ethical practices. This feature helps you gain insight into how HIPAA, law, and ethics relate to the performance of your duties.
- **Realistic ECG strips:** ECG rhythm strips have been provided for easy viewing and to make the task of learning the various dysrhythmias easier and more realistic. Activities and exercises throughout the program using these ECG rhythm strips provide for visual learners and improve understanding.

- **Chapter Summary and Review:** Once you have completed each chapter, take time to read the summary and complete the chapter review questions, which are presented in a variety of formats. These questions help you understand the content presented in each chapter.
- **Get Connected and the Online Learning Center:** The Get Connected activity directs you to the Online Learning Center (OLC) that accompanies the text/workbook. The OLC provides links for you to complete research and activities relative to the information presented in the chapter. You will also find other review activities and materials on the OLC to assist you in learning electrocardiography.
- **Chapter test:** Open the student CD to take a final test of your knowledge relative to each chapter. Review the material again with the Spin the Wheel game and then take the chapter test. You can print or e-mail your score to your instructor.

Instructor's Manual and Instructor CD

Look to the instructor's manual and the instructor CD for multiple resources to use while teaching *Electrocardiography for Health Care Personnel*. PowerPoint presentations for each chapter have Apply Your Knowledge questions at the end of each section and can be used for classroom presentation and discussion. An EZ-Test test bank that contains a variety of questions with graphics allows you to simply and easily create your own final or chapter exam. Also available are suggested classroom activities that will increase the interest level and comprehension of the text/workbook/CD material. Anticipatory set activities for each chapter help stimulate and enhance student learning as you begin each new topic. Curriculum suggestions provide information on how to use the materials based on your course length and depth. All media on the student CD are conveniently provided on the instructor CD for classroom presentations.

Guided Tour

Features to Help You Study and Learn

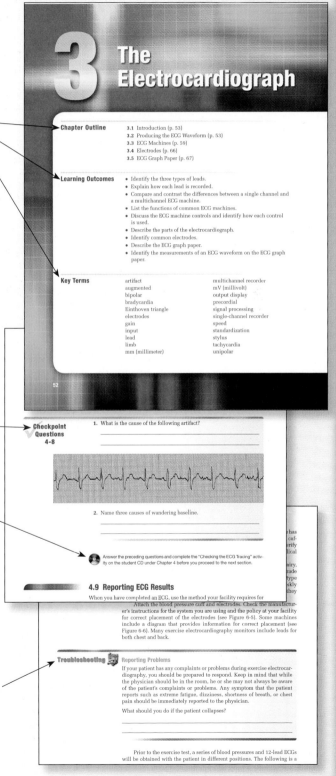

Chapter Outlines, Learning Outcomes, Key Terms, and an Introduction begin each chapter to introduce you to the chapter and help prepare you for the information that will be presented.

Checkpoint Questions are provided at the end of each section in the chapter to help you understand the information you just read.

CD-ROM references direct you to the interactive CD activity to further your review and practice the concepts presented in each section.

"The CD ROM is a great learning tool and is user friendly. The information on universal precautions is very important and not covered in other EKG texts." Sheri Melton, PhD, West Chester University

Troubleshooting exercises identify problems and situations that may arise on the job. You may be asked to answer a question about the situation.

Patient Education and Communication boxes give you helpful information communicating effectively—both orally and written—with patients.

"I have been examining textbooks for approximately eight years now and this ECG text provides students with the most complete and accurate information without overwhelming them." Donna Folmar, Belmont Technical College

Patients must be prepared for the ambulatory monitoring procedure both emotionally and physically. Many times the patient will be apprehensive. Children may be especially fearful. The first step in reducing the fear is to help them understand the procedure. Take time with the patient to explain each step of the procedure as you perform it. For children, be sure to explain in terms they can understand. Let the patient know it is normal to have some fear and allow the patient to express his or her feelings. Allow the patient to ask questions, and answer as completely as you can. If you do not know the answer, ask a licensed practitioner or your supervisor.

The patient should understand the physical requirements of the monitoring procedure. If the patient is male, he may have to have his chest shaved in order to place the electrodes. For both males and females, there may be some discomfort while the electrodes are in place. You should remind patients that during the procedure they should maintain all regular physical activities.

Patient Education & Communication — **Pediatric Patients**

Pediatric patients require special consideration when explaining the ambulatory monitoring procedure. Consider the child's age and use terms that he or she will understand. To decrease the child's potential anxieties and fears, allow the patient to touch the equipment prior to applying it. Be sure to instruct the parent as well.

Checkpoint Question 7-6

1. While answering questions for a patient, she asks something and you do not know the answer. What would you say?

Answer the preceding question and complete the "Preparing the Patient" activity on the student CD under Chapter 7 before you proceed to the next section.

Figure 3-12 Choose the right size and type of graph paper for the ECG machine you will be using.

3.4 Electrodes

Electrodes are sensors that are placed on a person's skin to pick up the electrical activity of the heart and conduct it to the ECG machine. The standard 12-lead ECG uses 10 electrodes. These electrodes come in a variety of types and are usually disposable. Reusable electrodes are essentially a thing of the past. If used, they however, do require care and maintenance.

Disposable Electrodes

Disposable electrodes are used because they reduce the possibility of cross-contamination and can be simply removed and discarded for easier cleanup (see Figure 3-12). The self-adhesive types stick easily to the patient's body. The gel is already applied so the electrodes will properly conduct the electrical impulses.

Safety and Infection Control boxes present tips and techniques for you to apply on the job.

Safety and Infection Control — **Do Not Mix Electrodes**

You should never mix two different types of electrodes. This could cause an inaccurate tracing, which could result in incorrect treatment for the patient.

Each disposable electrode is normally used on only one ECG. The only exception occurs when a second ECG is performed on the same patient immediately after the first and the electrodes are not disturbed. For example, if you are transferring a patient from an outpatient facility to a hospital, you should leave the electrodes in place for the emergency medical personnel. They will be recording one or more ECGs on the way to the hospital. If the electrodes stay on the patient's skin any longer than two sequential readings, the gel will dry out, resulting in inaccurate ECG tracings.

For hospitalized patients, longer-lasting silver electrodes are now available. These electrodes are used for patients who require multiple and frequent ECGs (serial ECGs). When serial ECGs are required, it is important

g, Remaining confusion

g a "stat"

HIPAA, Law, and Ethics boxes help you gain insight into necessary information related to the performance of your duties.

HIPAA, Law & Ethics — **What Is HIPAA?**

HIPAA or the Health Insurance Portability and Accountability Act was established in 1996 and passed into law in 2003. It is a national standard for the transfer of health care information. It established security and privacy for exchanging health data electronically and protects patient information. A patient's information cannot be shared among health care professionals unless it is for the patient's treatment. Fines may occur if you violate this law.

New technology has allowed for evaluation and monitoring of patients and their rhythms from a remote location. This is being referred to as an *e-ICU*. Patients are miles away being monitored by nurses for their heart rhythm and vital signs. This is in addition to the close monitoring done at the hospital.

Performing ECGs in Doctors' Offices and Ambulatory Care Clinics

A 12-lead ECG is a routine diagnostic test performed in almost any doctor's office or ambulatory care facility. It may be performed as part of a general or routine examination. This routine ECG provides a baseline tracing to be used for comparison if problems arise with a patient. The physician or trained expert looks for changes in a tracing that may indicate different types of health problems. Table 1-2 provides a complete list of conditions that may be diagnosed by an ECG. The procedure for performing a 12-lead ECG is discussed in Chapter 4.

Two other ECG-type tests that may be performed in an office include treadmill stress testing and the ambulatory monitor or **Holter monitor** testing (see Figure 1-4 and Figure 1-5).

The treadmill stress test, also known as exercise electrocardiography, is done to determine if the heart gets adequate blood flow during stress or exercise. While the stress test is being performed, the patient is attached to an ECG monitor as he or she is walking on the treadmill. The speed of the

ECG rhythm strips make the task of learning the various dysrhythmisa easier and more realistic.

"Practice ECG rhythm strips are key tool for practicing rhythm recognition. An excellent comprehensive textbook for the Electrocardiography student." Stephen Nardozzi, Westchester Community College

The patient who exhibits sinus bradycardia may or may not experience signs and symptoms of low cardiac output. When administering an ECG to a patient with a slow heart rate, it is important to observe for the symptoms of low cardiac output (see Table 5-2). Remember, though the patient may look all right, he or she can quickly experience difficulties with low cardiac output. When you observe symptoms of low cardiac output, report any findings to a licensed practitioner immediately. This rhythm may require drug administration or application of a pacemaker.

Sinus Tachycardia

Sinus tachycardia is a condition in which the sinoatrial node fires and the electrical impulse travels through the normal conduction pathway but the rate of impulse firing is faster than 100 beats per minute (see Figure 5-9).

Criteria for Classification

- *Rhythm:* The R-R interval and P-P interval will be equal and constant.
- *Rate:* Both the atrial and ventricular rates will be the same, between 100 and 150 beats per minute.

Figure 5-9 Sinus tachycardia.

1/12/07 12

Key points in the Chapter Summaries help you review what was just learned.

Chapter Summary

- The patient, the room, and the equipment must be properly prepared prior to performing an ECG.
- When a patient refuses an ECG, you should identify the cause, alleviate any fears, notify your supervisor, and document the refusal on the medical record.
- In order to place the electrodes properly for an ECG you must be able to locate anatomical landmarks including the midclavicular line, anterior axillary line, intercostal spaces, suprasternal notch, and the angle of Louis.
- Following standard precautions and performing hand hygiene are two ways to prevent infection during an ECG. In addition, isolation precautions may be used in a hospital or other in-patient health care facility.
- Maintain safety during an ECG by checking the plug and power cord, raising the bed to a working height, keeping the side rail up on the opposite side of the bed, and performing hand hygiene and wearing personal protective equipment, when necessary.
- To ensure HIPAA compliance when identifying a patient, you must use at least two patient identifiers, neither of which should be the patient's room number.
- Three types of artifact include somatic tremor caused by muscle movement, wandering baseline usually caused by improperly applied electrodes, or poor skin prep, and AC interference caused by some type of electrical interference.
- ECGs are recorded electronically and in paper fashion. Although they may be "read" by the machine, they must be provided promptly in a proper format to the practitioner who will be interpreting them.
- Single channel ECG tracings are cut and mounted for easy viewing and interpretation.
- During a pediatric ECG the chest lead V3 may need to be placed on the right side of the chest due to the small size of the chest.
- Many special patient considerations can occur during an ECG, such as for female patients, pregnant patients, amputees, and geriatric patients.
- Upon completion of an ECG the equipment must be cleaned and stored properly according to your facility guidelines and the manufacturer's recommendations.

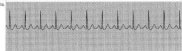

Chapter Review

Chapter Reviews consist of various methods of quizzing you. True/False, Multiple Choice, Matching, and Critical Thinking questions appeal to all types of learners.

At the end of each chapter, you will be directed to visit the Internet and the student CD to experience more interactive activities about the information you just learned.

The Matching

Match these terms with the correct definition. Place the appropriate letter on the line to the left of each term.

_____ 1. cardiovascular
_____ 2. electrocardiogram
_____ 3. arrhythmia
_____ 4. electro cardiology
_____ 5. electrocardiograph
_____ 6. defibrillator
_____ 7. AED

a. an instrument used to record the electrical activity of the heart
b. a tracing of the signal produced by the heart's electrical activity and used for diagnostic evaluation of the heart
c. the study of the heart's electrical activity
d. abnormal or absence of normal heartbeat, also known as dysrhythmia
e. used to analyze the heart rhythm and produce a shock if necessary
f. related to the heart and blood vessels (veins and arteries)
g. a machine that produces and sends an electrical shock to the heart that is intended to correct the abnormal electrical pattern of the heart

True/False

Read each statement and determine if it is true or false. Place a T or F on the line provided. For each of the false (F) statements, correct them to "make them true."

_____ 8. An ECG machine produces and records the electrical activity of the heart.
_____ 9. Standard precautions are guidelines written for health care providers to help prevent the spread of infection.
_____ 10. When performing an ECG, you should know the equipment, infection control principles, communication techniques, and safety guidelines.
_____ 11. A transtelephonic monitor transmits an ECG over the Internet.

Multiple Choice

Circle the correct answer.

12. Which of the following is *not* a reason that an ECG is performed?
   a. To determine how well the heart is pumping
   b. To determine if a person will experience a heart attack in the next month

Acknowledgments

Authors

Kathryn Booth: Thanks to all the reviewers that have spent time making sure this second edition is up-to-date. In addition, I would like to acknowledge McGraw-Hill for supporting this book into its second edition including Roxan Kinsey, Connie Kuhl, and Sheila Frank for their support and assistance. And a special acknowledgement to Patti, Tom, Cynthia, Jennifer, and Susan for all their time, attention and efforts in helping make this project a success.

Patricia DeiTos: I would like to acknowledge the members of the Inova Health system, who help to create and support the development of this textbook, the Inova Learning Network, who provided encouragement and lab space for photo opportunities. Also, acknowledge the members of the Inova Heart and Vascular Institute and Inova eICU for their assistance in obtaining photographs and video selections. Specifically, I would like to thank the managers for coordinating the photos and staff members willing to share their expertise and willingness to be photographed.

Thomas O'Brien: I would like to acknowledge Mr. David Rubin, President & CEO of Aerotel Medical Systems (1998) Ltd., 5 Hazoref St., Holon 58856, ISRAEL.

Consultants

Cynthia T. Vincent, MMS, PA-C
North Big Otter Clinic
Ivydale, West Virginia

Jennifer Childers MS PAC
Assistant Professor of Physician Assistant Studies
Alderson Broaddus College, Philippi, WV

Susan Hurley Findley, RN, MSN
Houston, TX

Reviewers

Second Edition

Emil P. Asdurian, MD
Bramson ORT College
Forest Hills, NY

Vanessa J. Austin, RMA, CAHI
Clarian Health Sciences Center,
  Medical Assistant
Indianapolis, IN

Rhonda J. Beck, NREMT-P
Central Georgia Technical College
Macon, GA

Nia Bullock, PhD
Miller-Motte Technical College
Cary, NC

Barbara S. Desch, LVN, CPC, AHI
San Joaquin Valley College Inc.
Visalia/Hanford Campus
Visalia, CA

Melissa L. Dulaney
MedVance Institute of Baton Rouge
Baton Rouge, LA

Mary Patricia English
Howard Community College
Columbia, MD

Michael Fisher, Program
    Director
Greenville Technical College
Greenville, SC

Donna L. Folmar
Belmont Technical College
St. Clairsville, OH

Anne Fox
Maric College
Carson, CA

James R. Fry, MS, PA-C
Marietta College
Marietta, OH

Michael Gallucci, MS, PT
Assistant Professor of Practice,
    Program in Physical
    Therapy
School of Public Health,
    New York Medical College
New York, NY

Jonathan I. Greenwald
Arapahoe Community College
Littleton, CO

Susie Laughter, BSN, RN
Cambridge Institute of Allied Health
Longwood, FL

Sheri A. Melton, PhD
West Chester University
West Chester, PA

Stephen J. Nardozzi
Westchester Community College
Valhalla, NY

David James Newton, NREMT-P
Dalton State College
Dalton, GA

R. Keith Owens
AB-Tech Community College
Asheville, NC

Douglas A. Paris, BS, NREMT-P
Greenville Technical College
Department of Emergency Medical
    Technology
Greenville, SC

David Rice, AA, BA, MA
Career College of Northern Nevada
Reno, NV

Dana M. Roessler, RN, BSN
Southeastern Technical College
Glennville, GA

Wayne A. Rummings, Sr.
Lenoir Community College
Kingston, NC

David Lee Sessoms, Jr., M.Ed.,
    CMA
Miller-Motte Technical College
Cary, NC

Mark A. Simpson, NREMT-P, RN,
    CCEMTP
Director of EMS
Northwest-Shoals Community
    College
Muscle Shoals, AL

Linda M. Thompson, MS, RRT
Madison Area Technical College
Madison, WI

Dyan Whitlow Underhill,
    MHA, BS
Miller-Motte Technical College
Cary, NC

Eddy van Hunnik, PhD
Gibbs College Boston
Boston, MA

Danielle Schortzmann Wilken
Goodwin College
East Hartford, CT

Stacey F. Wilson, MT/PBT (ASCP),
    CMA
Cabarrus College of Health
    Sciences
Concord, NC

Roger G. Wootten
Northeast Alabama Community
    College
Rainsville, AL

First Edition

Civita Allard
Mohawk Valley Community
    College
Utica, NY

Vicki Barclay
West Kentucky Technical College
Paducah, KY

Nina Beaman
Bryant and Stratton College
Richmond, VA

Cheryl Bell
Sanz School
Washington, DC

Lucy Della Rosa
Concorde Career Institute

Lauderdale Lakes, FL

Myrna Lanier
Tulsa Community College
Tulsa, OK

Debra Shafer
Blair College
Colorado Springs, CO

Role of the Electrocardiographer

1

Learning Outcomes

- Explain what an ECG is and its importance in medicine.
- Discuss the history of obtaining and using the ECG.
- Describe career opportunities for an electrocardiographer.
- List the uses of the ECG in the hospital, in the doctor's office or ambulatory clinic, or outside of a health care facility.
- Identify the skills and knowledge needed to perform an ECG.
- Define troubleshooting and explain its importance to you as a health care professional.

Key Terms

angioplasty	electrocardiology
arrhythmia	galvanometer
automatic external defibrillator (AED)	health care providers
	Holter monitor
cardiovascular	myocardial infarction (MI) (heart
Code Blue	attack)
coronary vascular disease (CVD)	pacemaker
defibrillator	technician
electrocardiogram (ECG)	technologist
electrocardiograph	telemetry

1.1 Introduction

The number one cause of death in America every year since 1918 is **cardiovascular** disease or a disease of the heart and blood vessels. Approximately 2500 Americans die every day because of **coronary vascular disease (CVD)**, which is narrowing of the blood vessels surrounding the heart causing a reduction of blood flow to the heart. Cardiovascular disease claims more lives than the next four leading causes of death all together. These other causes include cancer, respiratory diseases, accidents, and diabetes. Unbelievably, one out of every three American adults has some form of CVD. You may know someone who has hypertension (high blood pressure) or other heart conditions. Maybe someone you know has had an MI (myocardial infarction, or heart attack). See Table 1-1 for more information on ways to reduce or prevent heart disease, stroke, or heart attack.

An instrument used to produce the ECG tracings, which allows the heart's electrical activity to be studied, is known as an **electrocardiograph.** The machine records the electrical activity within the heart. It is used to produce an electrical (*electro*) tracing (*graph*) of the heart (*cardio*). This tracing is known as an **electrocardiogram,** or ECG. The standard ECG machine has lead wires that are attached to a patient's chest to produce the electrical tracing (see Figure 1-1).

Performing the actual ECG procedure is not difficult; however, it must be performed competently. The tracing of the electrical current of the heart must be accurate because it is used to make decisions about a patient's care.

TABLE 1-1   Ways to Reduce or Prevent Heart Disease, Stroke, or Heart Attack

The American Heart Association now recommends that you watch your ABCs:

A. Avoid tobacco.
1. Stop smoking. A smoker's risk is twice that of a nonsmoker. Even exposure to environmental tobacco smoke (secondhand smoke, passive smoking) may increase the risk of heart disease.
2. Decrease stress.
3. Maintain healthy blood pressure. Lower blood pressure to keep the numbers down and stay down. The goal is a blood pressure of less than 120/80 mm Hg.
4. Maintain healthy blood cholesterol. Cholesterol will cause the fat to be lodged in your arteries, which will sooner or later cause a heart attack or stoke. It is important to keep the total cholesterol less than 200 mg/dL.

B. Be more active.
1. Increase physical activity. Goal is to increase physical activities on most days of the week to 30 to 60 minutes of physical activity. Increase in activity will decrease the following:
   a. Stress
   b. High blood pressure
   c. High blood cholesterol
   d. Obesity

C. Choose good nutrition. Maintain a well-balanced diet, which helps to decrease the following:
1. Alcohol consumption
2. Stress
3. High blood pressure
4. High blood cholesterol
5. Diabetes
6. Obesity

Adapted from the American Heart Association

Figure 1-1 A 12-lead ECG machine is attached to the patient's chest, arms, and legs using electrodes and leads. It records the electrical tracing of the heart.

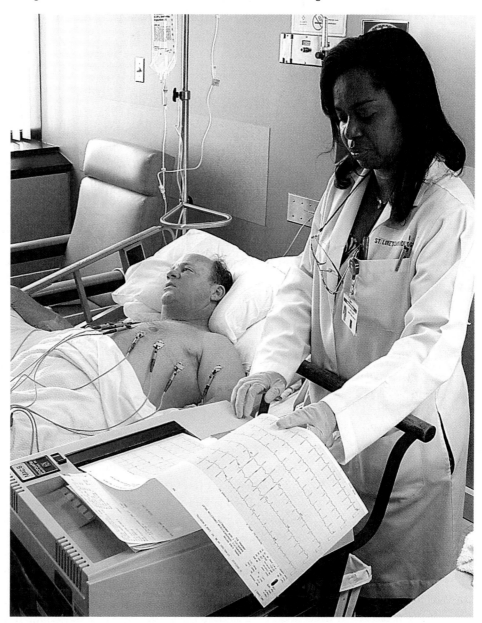

An inaccurate tracing could result in a wrong decision about the patient's medication or treatment. These decisions could result in a negative outcome for the patient.

An ECG may be performed for any of the following reasons:

- To check for problems with the flow of electricity through the heart
- To diagnose changes in the heart rhythm
- To check for abnormalities before surgery
- To assist in evaluating a person's health after age 40 during a complete physical exam
- To monitor or evaluate individuals with heart conditions
- To monitor or evaluate effectiveness of cardiac treatments such as medications

Checkpoint Question 1-1

1. What is the leading cause of death in the United States?

_____

_____

1.2 History of the ECG

Knowing the history of obtaining electrical tracings of the heart will help you better understand the reasons ECGs are performed and their importance in medicine. As early as 1676, scientists made the discovery that animals generate electricity. In 1887, an English physician, Dr. Augusta D. Waller (1856–1922), was the first to show that electrical currents are produced during the beating of the human heart and can be recorded. Dr. Waller was credited with having performed the first electrocardiogram on a human.

Safety and Infection Control

Electricity and the ECG

An ECG does not produce electricity; it only records the electrical activity of the heart. It is a safe and harmless procedure.

Wilhelm Einthoven (1860–1927), a Dutch physiologist, continued the development of the ECG. He developed the first practical **galvanometer,** an instrument used to detect electrocardiograph waves. In 1903, Einthoven invented the first electrocardiograph. Einthoven's instrument introduced the field of **electrocardiology,** and he won the Nobel Prize in Physiology or Medicine in 1924 for the significance of his invention.

Other scientists extended the work of Einthoven. Sir Thomas Lewis of London (1881–1945) studied how the ECG related to cardiac **arrhythmias** (abnormal heartbeats). He formed the basis for much of the current knowledge about the ECG. In 1918, an American physician, James B. Herrick, showed that an abnormal tracing and physical symptoms could indicate a **myocardial infarction (MI),** also known as a heart attack.

Advancements in technology have brought today's modern ECG machines. Computer interpretation of the ECG tracing is common. Currently, computer technology continues to improve the availability and speed of computer interpretation and quickly communicates this information to a health care professional. An ECG machine is now as small as a wristwatch. With the use of digital information, health care professionals are able to monitor patients from remote locations miles away. Nurses and physicians can monitor the patients through cameras and ECG readings and other vital sign measurements to assist the health care professional working at the bedside.

Checkpoint Question 1-2

1. Who is credited with having performed the first ECG on a human?

_____

_____

Answer the preceding question and complete the "History of the ECG" activity on the student CD under Chapter 1 before you proceed to the next section.

1.3 Role of an Electrocardiographer

Electrocardiography is an expanding career field. Many health care professionals are trained to record or monitor the heart's electrical activity. These include physicians, nurse practitioners, physician assistants, nurses, paramedics, medical assistants, trained nursing assistants, and emergency medical technicians, though this list is not inclusive. With the changing health care field, other health care employees such as respiratory or radiology personnel are also learning to perform ECGs to improve health care delivery in a variety of health care settings.

Health care personnel who are proficient at recording an ECG can expect to increase their employability and advance their careers. In addition, there are career opportunities for individuals who may want to specialize in the field of electrocardiography. These include but are not limited to the ECG technician, the ECG monitoring technician, and the cardiovascular technologist.

An electrocardiograph (ECG) **technician** is an individual who records the ECG and prepares the report for the physician. ECG technicians should be able to determine if the tracing is accurate and recognize abnormalities caused by interference during the recording procedure. Most ECG technicians are employed in hospitals. They may also work in medical offices, cardiac centers, cardiac rehabilitation centers, and other health care facilities. In some large hospitals, the ECG technician works in the home health care branch. He or she takes the ECG machine to the patient's home, records the ECG, and gives, sends, or telecommunicates the report to the physician for interpretation. With the development of multiple tests to evaluate the heart, the ECG technician who obtains continuing education can expect a rewarding career.

ECG monitor technicians view and evaluate the electrical tracings of patients' hearts on an oscilloscope (see Figure 1-2). ECG monitor technicians are employed at hospitals or other inpatient facilities where patients are attached to continuous or **telemetry** monitors. The main responsibility of an ECG monitor technician is to view the ECG tracings and, if an abnormal heart rhythm occurs, alert the health care professional who can treat the abnormality. ECG monitor technicians are required to understand the various heart rhythms and recognize abnormal ones. ECG monitor technicians must be able to evaluate the ECG tracing. They may also be asked to perform other duties such as maintaining patient records and recording ECGs.

If you enjoy the field of electrocardiology and want to advance your skills or education, you may choose to be a cardiovascular **technologist.** Technologists require more extensive training than technicians. They may assist physicians with invasive cardiovascular diagnostic tests such as **angioplasty,** heart surgery, or implantation of electronic, artificial **pacemakers.** Another specialization for cardiovascular technologists is performing ultrasounds on the blood vessels. Ultrasound equipment transmits sound waves and then collects the echoes to form an image on a screen. As part of their duties, cardiovascular technologists may also perform ECGs.

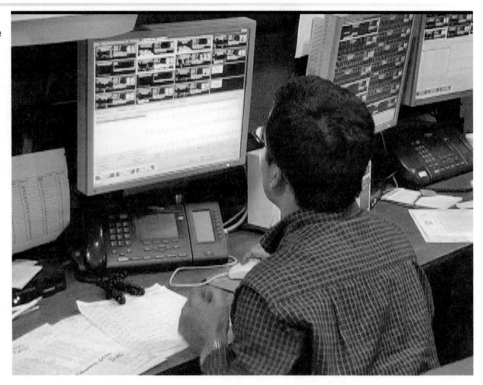

Figure 1-2 An ECG monitor technician may be responsible for monitoring multiple patient ECG tracings.

Checkpoint Question 1-3

1. An ECG technician's role includes the following:

_____

_____

Answer the preceding question and complete the "Role of an Electrocardiographer" activity on the student CD under Chapter 1 before you proceed to the next section.

1.4 How ECGs Are Used

Health care providers study the ECG tracing to determine many things about the patient's heart. They look for changes from the normal ECG tracing or from the first ECG tracing, which provides a baseline for comparison of subsequent ECGs performed. The American Heart Association recommends that individuals over the age of 40 have an ECG done annually as part of a complete physical. This baseline tracing assists the physician in diagnosing abnormalities of the heart. A sample of a normal tracing is shown in Figure 1-3. We discuss normal and abnormal ECG tracings in Chapter 2 and Chapter 5 of this text.

The ECG tracing is recorded using a variety of ECG machines and can be performed in a number of health care settings. These include acute care settings such as hospitals, ambulatory care settings such as clinics or doctors' offices, and even outside of a health care facility. Emergency personnel routinely perform ECGs during emergencies. An ECG tracing can also be transmitted over the telephone, mobile, or Internet from a person's home or

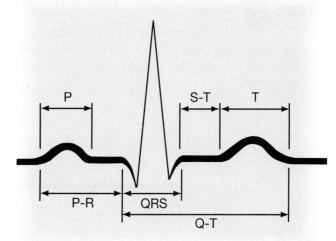

Figure 1-3 A normal ECG tracing is a straight line with upward and downward spikes or deflections, that indicate electrical activity within the heart.

other remote location. The type of ECG tracing produced depends upon the setting and the type of ECG machine used to record.

In the Hospital (Acute Care)

A 12-lead ECG is one of the most commonly used ECGs in the hospital setting. A 12-lead ECG provides a tracing of the electrical activity in the patient's heart at the exact time the ECG tracing is done. In the hospital, a 12-lead ECG is done as a routine procedure or during an emergency such as a **Code Blue.** An emergency ECG may be referred to as "stat," meaning immediately. These are done when a patient experiences chest pain or has a change in his or her cardiac rhythm. Routine ECGs are usually obtained in the early morning so they are available for the physician to review when he or she does patient rounds. Routine ECGs are also frequently done before surgery. Both routine or stat ECGs must be performed safely and with accuracy. The tracing you record will provide critical information about the patient. An inaccurate tracing could result in misdiagnosis, incorrect medications being administered, or other serious outcomes.

Another use of the ECG tracing in the hospital is in continuous monitoring. The purpose of continuous monitoring is to check the pattern of the electrical activity of the patient's heart over time. During continuous monitoring, electrodes are attached to the patient's chest and the tracing is viewed on an oscilloscope. Patients on continuous monitoring are usually in an intensive care unit (ICU), coronary care unit or cardiac care unit (CCU), surgical intensive care unit (SICU), or even an emergency room (ER). Some continuous monitors can also monitor the vital signs and the oxygen level in the blood. Continuous monitoring is also done routinely during surgery.

Another type of continuous monitoring done in a hospital is known as *telemetry monitoring.* Telemetry monitors are small boxes with electrodes and lead wires attached to the chest. The monitor is usually housed in a case and is attached to the patient so he or she can move about. The ECG tracing is transmitted to a central location for evaluation. When several patients are on a telemetry unit, the tracings of all the patients are recorded on multiple oscilloscopes at the nursing or patient care station.

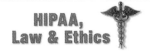
New technology has allowed for evaluation and monitoring of patients and their rhythms from a remote location. This is being referred to as an *e-ICU*. Patients are miles away being monitored by nurses for their heart rhythm and vital signs. This is in addition to the close monitoring done at the hospital.

Performing ECGs in Doctors' Offices and Ambulatory Care Clinics

A 12-lead ECG is a routine diagnostic test performed in almost any doctor's office or ambulatory care facility. It may be performed as part of a general or routine examination. This routine ECG provides a baseline tracing to be used for comparison if problems arise with a patient. The physician or trained expert looks for changes in a tracing that may indicate different types of health problems. Table 1-2 provides a complete list of conditions that may be diagnosed by an ECG. The procedure for performing a 12-lead ECG is discussed in Chapter 4.

Two other ECG-type tests that may be performed in an office include treadmill stress testing and the ambulatory monitor or **Holter monitor** testing (see Figure 1-4 and Figure 1-5).

The treadmill stress test, also known as exercise electrocardiography, is done to determine if the heart gets adequate blood flow during stress or exercise. While the stress test is being performed, the patient is attached to an ECG monitor as he or she is walking on the treadmill. The speed of the treadmill can be varied to measure how this might "stress" the heart. The

TABLE 1-2   Conditions Evaluated by the ECG

- Disorders in heart rate or rhythm and the conduction system
- Presence of electrolyte imbalance
- Condition of the heart prior to defibrillation
- Damage assessment during and after a myocardial infarction (heart attack)
- Symptoms related to cardiovascular disorders such as weakness, chest pain, or shortness of breath
- Diagnosis of certain drug toxicity
- Diagnosis of metabolic disorders such as hyper- or hypokalemia, hyper- or hypocalcemia, hyper- or hypothyroidism, acidosis, and alkalosis
- Heart condition prior to surgery for individuals at risk for undiagnosed or asymptomatic heart disease
- Damage assessment following blunt or penetrating chest trauma or changes after trauma or injury to the brain or spinal cord
- Assessment of the effects of cardiotoxic or antiarrhythmic therapy
- Suspicion of congenital heart disease
- Pacemaker function

ECG tracing is recorded and analyzed for changes during the exercise. A physician should always be present during this procedure. The stress test is frequently ordered because it is a safe, noninvasive, inexpensive, and reliable method of measuring the heart's condition if a problem is suspected by the physician. We discuss the stress test in more detail in Chapter 6.

A Holter monitor is a small box that is strapped to a patient's waist or shoulder to monitor the heart for 24 to 48 hours during a patient's normal daily activity. After the monitoring period, the patient returns to the office for the monitor to be removed. The ambulatory monitor is usually a small

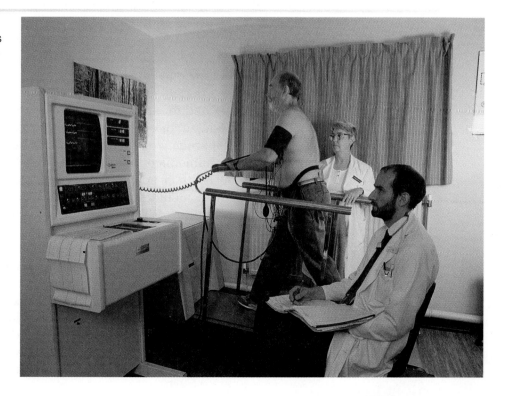

Figure 1-4   This patient is performing a treadmill stress test, also known as exercise electrocardiography. During the exercise, the patient's heart, blood pressure, and oxygen use are being monitored.

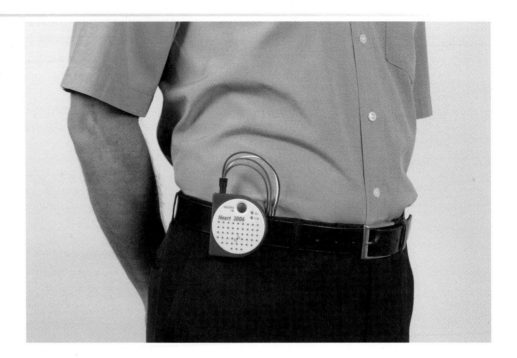

Figure 1-5 The Holter or ambulatory monitor allows the patient to participate in routine daily activities while the electrical activity of the heart is being recorded.

tape recorder or digital disc. When the recording is finished, it is examined with a special instrument called a scanner. The ECG tracing is then analyzed and interpreted by the physician. Some patients can connect these monitors to a computer where the information can be e-mailed to the physician. We discuss the ambulatory monitor in detail in Chapter 7.

Outside of a Health Care Facility

Outside of a health care facility, the ECG is a valuable tool used during a cardiac emergency such as a myocardial infarction. Emergency medical technicians and paramedics are equipped with portable ECG machines that can produce an ECG tracing at the site of the emergency. Whether the patient is at home, in a car, or in a crowded football stadium, emergency personnel can monitor and trace the electrical activity of the heart. Figure 1-6 shows one example of a portable ECG machine. In an emergency setting, the tracing can be evaluated for an abnormal ECG pattern. It is either transmitted back to the physician for evaluation or assessed by the emergency medical personnel at the scene. An abnormal pattern, such as for sudden cardiac arrest, requires immediate treatment; the patient becomes unresponsive, which leads to death if not treated within minutes. Treatment for these abnormal rhythms includes use of a **defibrillator** and/or administration of cardiac medications. When the heart is in this chaotic rhythm of ventricular fibrillation or pulseless ventricular tachycardia, the heart must be "defibrillated" quickly. The survival rate of the victim decreases 7% to 10% for every minute a normal heartbeat is not restored. A defibrillator produces an electrical shock to the heart that is intended to correct the heart's electrical pattern. A defibrillator is commonly used in emergencies such as a Code Blue in the hospital or other care facilities or at the site of the emergency by appropriate personnel.

Automatic external defibrillators (AEDs) have enabled lay rescuers to help a patient with sudden cardiac arrest (see Figure 1-7). AEDs are

Figure 1-6 This portable ECG monitor is transported to the scene during a cardiac emergency and is attached to the patient. The ECG tracing is recorded and viewed by the emergency personnel. In addition, the tracing can be transmitted to the hospital, where a physician can evaluate and determine the necessary drugs and treatment for the patient based upon the heart rhythm viewed and the report from the emergency personnel.

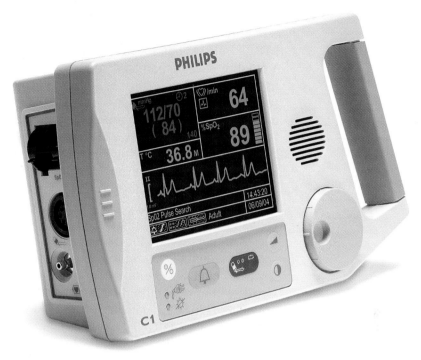

available in public and/or private places where large numbers of people gather or live or are kept by people who are at high risk for heart attacks. An AED is a lightweight, portable device that recognizes an abnormal rhythm and determines if the rhythm is considered a "shockable rhythm." The equipment

Figure 1-7 Automatic external defibrillators (AEDs) can reverse an abnormal heart rhythm and increase the survival rate of myocardial infarction victims. They can be found in public places and require minimal training to operate.

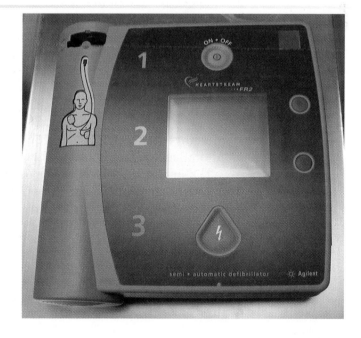

is *only* placed on patients who are unresponsive (not able to be aroused) to stimulation and have no evidence of breathing or a pulse. AEDs will only shock the rhythms of ventricular fibrillation or ventricular tachycardia that do not produce a heartbeat. These rhythms are discussed in Chapter 5. When the machine recognizes other rhythms that cause the patient to be unresponsive, the AED recommends beginning CPR.

Once the equipment is placed on the patient's bare chest, the machine will either automatically analyze or require the operator to push the "ANALYZE" button. The machine will analyze the rhythm to determine if it is a rhythm that responds with an electric shock through the chest to the heart. Once it has positively identified the abnormal rhythm, the machine will indicate that a "SHOCK IS ADVISED." All persons next to the patient must move back and not touch the patient. One person will then announce "I'm clear, you're clear, we are all clear" and press the shock button. After the shock has been provided, the rescuers continue administering CPR until the patient wakes up, the machine indicates to defibrillate again, or specially trained health care professionals take over. These new machines now make it possible for laypersons to perform defibrillation safely. The AED is being viewed as a necessary piece of equipment—similar to a fire extinguisher.

Another use of the ECG tracing outside of a health care facility is through telemedicine. In telemedicine, ECG tracings are communicated to the physician via the telephone or digital system. *Transtelephonic monitoring* means transmitted (*trans*) over the telephone (*telephonic*). The improvements in solid-state digital technology have expanded transtelephonic transmission of ECG data and enhanced the accuracy of software-based analysis systems. Digital monitoring allows for ECG data to be recorded with a personal computer and then transmitted over the Internet to the health care facility. Transtelephonic monitoring requires a licensed practitioner to read and evaluate the reading, whereas the digital monitoring provides a report that is validated by the licensed practitioner.

Both of these types of monitoring evaluate the ECG tracing of a patient over time. The two types of ambulatory monitoring methods are useful for patients with symptoms of heart disease that did not occur while they were in the health care facility. The recorded monitoring can be accomplished with magnetic tape (transtelephonic) or digital (computerized) that are used for up to 30 days. A transtelephonic monitor is placed on a telephone mouthpiece, and the ECG is transmitted to a health care facility on specific days through the monitoring (see Figure 1-8). Individuals using a transtelephonic monitor must understand when and how to record and send a transmission. A digital monitor requires the individual to be able to use a computer and understand how to send a transmission. Depending upon which equipment your facility uses, you may be required to teach the patient how to use the monitor. Become familiar with the type of monitor used at your facility.

There are two specific types of telemedicine monitors. One monitors the heart continuously, and the other records the ECG tracing when the patient is having symptoms. Continuous telemedicine monitoring is programmed to record the ECG tracing constantly. It is useful to record the ECG tracing before, during, and after a patient has symptoms. These symptoms may include chest pain, shortness of breath, dizziness, or palpitations. This type of monitor is a small device that attaches to the patient's chest with two electrodes. The smallest monitor available is about the size and shape of a beeper.

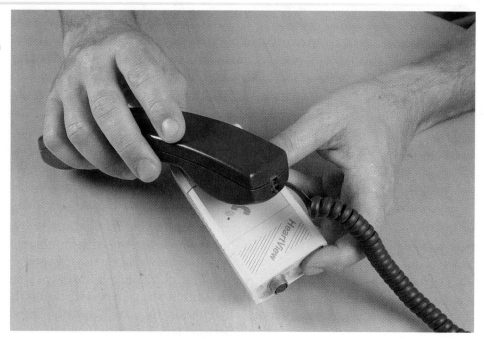

Figure 1-8 Transtelephonic monitors are connected to a telephone at a remote location and the ECG tracing is transmitted and viewed at a central location for interpretation.

Symptom-based telemedicine monitoring is in the form of either a handheld or a wristwatch device. The handheld type has electrode feet that are pressed against the patient's chest after symptoms occur. Currently, one type is as small as a credit card and can be carried in a pocket or wallet. The wristwatch type monitor is worn on the left arm at all times. The patient must turn on this type of monitor when symptoms begin.

Telemedicine monitoring is generally used to evaluate artificial pacemaker functioning. In addition, monitors are sometimes given to patients after an emergency room visit. If the patient has symptoms of cardiac problems but is not admitted to the hospital, a physician will often give the patient a monitor to record an ECG when the symptoms recur. It is less expensive to give patients a monitor to take home than to admit them to the hospital.

Checkpoint Questions 1-4

1. A 12-lead ECG can be obtained by an electrocardiographer in which health care venues?

   _____

   _____

2. An automatic external defibrillator (AED) is used to treat what conditions?

   _____

   _____

 Answer the preceding questions and complete the "How ECGs Are Used" activity on the student CD under Chapter 1 before you proceed to the next section.

1.5 What You Need to Know to Perform an ECG

In order to perform an ECG, you should become familiar with the procedure and the ECG machine. You must have the ability to lift and move the patient, if necessary. You need to be able to transport and operate the ECG machine. In addition, you must understand basic principles of safety and infection control, patient education and communication, and law and ethics. Being able to troubleshoot problems or situations that arise during the procedure is also essential.

Equipment

Knowing how to use the equipment is part of performing an ECG. You must be able to transport, operate, maintain, and store the ECG equipment used at your facility. There are many different machines available to perform an ECG, and directions provided by the manufacturer are an important source of information. Many ECG machines have reference cards or instructions posted in a convenient place on or with the equipment. Refer to these printed materials when performing an ECG. Although all ECG machines are similar, you should become familiar with the particular machine you are using. You should always perform at least one or two practice ECGs before using any machine on a patient. Since an ECG is noninvasive, you can practice on a volunteer, friend, co-worker, or fellow student.

Safety

When performing health care procedures, you must always maintain the safety of yourself and the patient. General safety guidelines should be followed at all times. Certain safety precautions specific to performing the ECG procedure should also be followed. These specific precautions are discussed in more detail in Chapter 4.

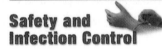
Safety and Infection Control

Guidelines

Follow safety and infection control guidelines at all times when working in a health care facility and performing an ECG.

Infection Control

Preventing the spread of infection is an essential part of providing health care and performing an ECG. This is for your safety as well as the safety of your patients. The Centers for Disease Control and Prevention (CDC) have implemented two levels of precautions to prevent infections—standard precautions and isolation precautions.

Standard precautions include a combination of hand hygiene and wearing gloves when there is a possibility of exposure to blood and body fluids, nonintact skin, or mucous membranes (see Figure 1-9). Standard precautions include the major features of universal precautions but apply to blood, all body fluids, secretions, and excretions except sweat, regardless of whether or not they contain visible blood, nonintact skin, and mucous membranes. Universal precautions apply to blood and any other body fluids *only* if they

Figure 1-9 The use of an alcohol-base rub on hands without visible soilage is a recommended technique for preventing infection.

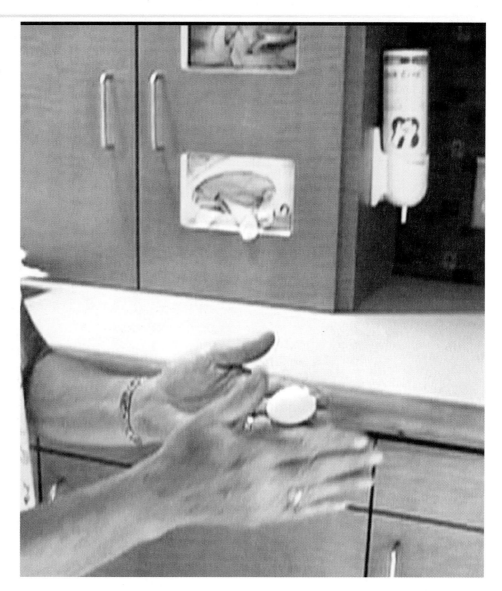

contain visible blood. Standard precautions reduce the risk of transmission of microorganisms from both recognized and unrecognized sources of infection. In addition to hand hygiene and wearing gloves, practices may include the use of a gown, mask, and eye protection (see Figure 1-10). In addition, the CDC advises that health care workers should not wear artificial nails, as workers are more likely to harbor gram-negative pathogens on their fingertips than are those with natural nails, both before and after handwashing. Natural nails should be no more than one-fourth inch long.

The second level includes *isolation precautions*, which are based on how the infectious agent is transmitted. Isolation precautions are

1. airborne precautions that require special air handling, ventilation, and additional respiratory protection (HEPA or N95 respirators);
2. droplet precautions requiring mucous membrane protection (goggles and masks); and
3. contact precautions requiring gloves and gowns for direct skin-to-skin contact or for contact with contaminated linen, equipment, and so on.

Figure 1-10 Personal protection equipment (PPE) is used to reduce the risk of transmission of infection. PPE includes items such as gloves, mask, gown, and eye protection.

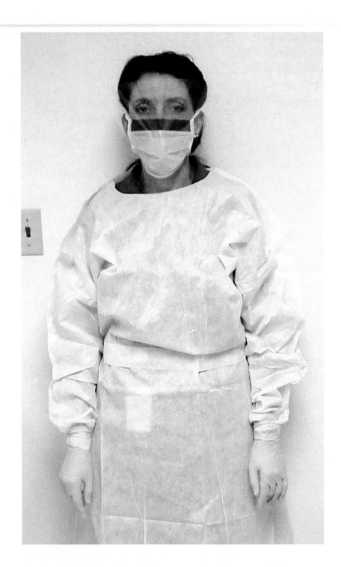

Standard precautions are practiced in all employment situations in which exposure to blood or body fluids is likely. Isolation precautions are used less often and only with patients who have specific infections. When isolation precautions are in place for a patient during an ECG, you will be required to follow the specific guidelines for the type of precautions implemented. Table 1-3 provides a list of standard precautions that should be practiced when recording an ECG.

Patient Education and Communication

Communicating with your patients is key to successfully recording an ECG. You must develop a positive relationship and atmosphere to reduce apprehension and anxiety during an ECG. You can reduce the patient's fears and make the ECG a positive experience by developing a helpful relationship with your patient and practicing effective communication techniques. Clearly explaining the procedure and answering questions are essential for good patient communication. Maintain a friendly, confident manner while interacting with your patient. Your patient will be more cooperative if he or she trusts that you are competent to perform your job.

TABLE 1-3   **Standard Precautions Related to Electrocardiography**

Hand Hygiene
- Wash your hands after touching blood, body fluids, secretions, excretions, and contaminated items.
- Wash your hands before putting on gloves and after removing gloves.
- Wash your hands between patient contacts.
- Wash your hands between tasks and procedures on the same person.
- Use Alcohol-based hand rub if you have no visible soilage.

Gloves
- Wear gloves when touching blood, body fluids, secretions, excretions, and contaminated items.
- Wear gloves when touching mucous membranes and nonintact skin.
- Change gloves between procedures and patients.
- Change gloves after contacting materials that are highly contaminated.
- Remove gloves promptly after use.
- Remove gloves before touching uncontaminated surfaces or items.
- Wash your hands immediately after glove removal.

Masks, Eye Protection, and Face Shields
- Masks, eye protection, and face shields protect the mucous membranes of the mouth, eyes, and nose from splashes and sprays.
- Wear mask, eye protection, and face shields during procedures and tasks that are likely to cause splashes or sprays of blood, body fluids, secretions, and excretions.

Gowns
- Gowns protect the skin and clothing.
- Wear a gown during procedures and activities that are likely to cause splashes or sprays of blood, body fluids, secretions, or excretions.
- Remove a soiled gown promptly.
- Wash your hands immediately after gown removal.

Equipment
- Equipment may be soiled with blood, body fluids, secretions, and excretions.
- Handle used equipment carefully.
- Prevent skin and mucous membrane exposure and clothing contamination.
- Reusable equipment must be cleaned, disinfected, or sterilized before it is used on another person.
- Discard single-use equipment promptly.

Environmental Control
- Follow facility procedures for the routine care, cleaning, and disinfection of surfaces. This includes environmental surfaces, nonmovable equipment, and other frequently touched surfaces.

Occupational Health and Bloodborne Pathogens
- Use resuscitation devices for mouth-to-barrier resuscitation.

Helping the patient understand the procedure and follow instructions is essential to performing any ECG procedure. When explaining the procedure, use simple terms and speak slowly and distinctly. Encourage the patient to ask questions and repeat the instructions. This process will help ensure patient understanding.

In addition, in your role as a multiskilled health care professional, you will need to be able to work in a variety of situations as a team member and be able to resolve conflicts. As with any job, you should continue to improve in your performance through further education and practice.

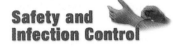

Safety and Infection Control

Hand Hygiene

Proper hand hygiene is the single most important thing you can do to prevent the spread of infection. Handwashing or the use of an alcohol-based rub on hands without visible soilage should be practiced between patients and procedures and before and after the use of gloves.

Legal and Ethical Issues

As a multiskilled health care professional, you must understand some legal and ethical considerations of patient care. Laws are rules of conduct that are enforced by a controlling authority such as the government. An unlawful act can result in loss of your job, a fine, or other penalty such as time in jail. Ethics are concerned with standards of behavior and concepts of right and wrong. They are based upon moral values that are formed through the influence of the family, culture, and society. Unethical acts result in poor job evaluations or job loss. When comparing law and ethics, you should understand that illegal acts are always unethical but unethical acts are not always illegal.

Patient Education & Communication

Improving Communication

When speaking to a patient who is hard of hearing, look directly at the patient and speak slowly and distinctly. The patient may be able to read your lips. When your patient speaks another language, you may want to ask an interpreter or family member to assist you with communication, thus reducing apprehension and anxiety.

Protecting Patient Information: HIPAA

Patient information has always been considered to be confidential or private. In 1996, the Health Insurance Portability and Accountability Act (HIPAA) was established in response to information that was being transferred electronically for medical transactions. This Act establishes a national standard for electronic health care transactions and also for providers, health plans, and employers. It was to ensure that the widespread use of electronic data was limited and secured. The patient can specify who is able to see information and what information is protected. A patient's information can only be sent and viewed when specific to insurance payments and further medical treatment with a consulting health care professional. A patient's information cannot be shared among health care professionals unless it is for the patient's treatment.

Practicing Ethics

Many professions have a code of ethics. These are standards of behavior or conduct as defined by the professional group. As a health care professional, you must follow the standards of behavior or code of ethics set forth by your profession and place of employment. The following are some basic ethics you should practice.

Confidentiality is an essential part of patient care. You may collect information about a patient for use during his or her care and treatment; however, this information should not be made public. Confidentiality is a basic right of every patient. You should not speak about your patients or allow information about your patients to be heard or seen by anyone other than those caring for them. A breach in confidentiality is unethical, illegal, and a violation of HIPAA.

Patients should be treated with respect and dignity. You should respect the privacy of patients at all times. Avoid exposing your patient's body when performing any procedure by closing the door, pulling the curtain, and/or draping the patient.

Practicing ethics also includes professionalism, respect, and cooperation. You should maintain professionalism by continuing your education and training in order to provide the highest level of care for your patient. You should respect your patient's beliefs, values, and morals; and you should work cooperatively with your co-workers and supervisors at all times.

Legal Issues You Should Know

Medical professional liability means that a health care professional is legally responsible for his or her performance. Health care professionals can be held accountable for performing unlawful acts, performing legal acts improperly, or simply failing to perform an act when they should. For example, if you find a patient's wallet after he or she leaves and you decide to keep it, this is an illegal act. While you are assisting with a treadmill stress test, if you report the blood pressure results incorrectly, resulting in the patient having a severe heart attack, this is performing a legal act improperly. If you decide to take a break when you are supposed to be monitoring a patient's heart rhythm and during the time you are gone the patient experiences an abnormal heart rhythm resulting in death from lack of prompt treatment, you have failed to perform your duties as required.

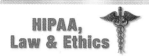

HIPAA, Law & Ethics

Keep Information Private

The patient's chart or computer screen with patient data should not be left out or open in an area where other patients or visitors may be able to view it. This is a breach of confidentiality and HIPAA.

You will be speaking and writing about patients as part of your job as an electrocardiographer. You should never speak defamatory words about patients even when they upset you. Making derogatory remarks about a patient—or anyone else—that jeopardizes his or her reputation or means of livelihood is called *slander*. Slander is an illegal and unethical act that could cause you to lose your job. If you write defamatory words, this is known as *libel*, which is also illegal and unethical.

Medical care and treatment must be documented as part of the medical record. The medical record can be used in court as evidence in a medical professional liability case. To protect yourself legally and provide continuity of patient care, you should include complete information in the medical record. See Table 1-4 for a complete list of the necessary information to document on the medical record.

Whatever ECG procedure you are performing, the patient must agree or consent to having the procedure done. Implied consent is between the patient and health care professional such as a physician in an office. For example, when a patient requests care and comes to the physician's office, he or she is agreeing to be treated by the physician. This is *implied* consent. When a patient agrees to the ECG procedure, this is also implied consent.

Certain diagnostic procedures, including a treadmill stress test, require *informed* consent. The patient must understand the procedure and its associated risks, alternative procedures and their risks, and the potential risks to the patient if he or she refuses treatment. Informed consent requires the patient to sign a consent form.

Troubleshooting

When caring for patients and recording an ECG, you may experience a variety of problems. These problems may stem from the patient's condition, patient communication, equipment failure, or other complications. While performing an ECG, you may need to troubleshoot actual or potential complications during the procedure. Troubleshooting requires critical thinking. Critical thinking is the process of thinking through the situation or problem and making a decision to solve it. Let us say that you are about to perform an ECG and the patient refuses to let you attach the lead wires. As part of troubleshooting, you ask the patient why he or she is refusing. The patient

TABLE 1-4 **Required Entries for Medical Records Related to ECG**

- Patient identification, including full name, social security number, birth date, full address and telephone number, marital status, and place of employment, if applicable
- Patient's medical history
- Dates and times of all appointments, admissions, discharge, and diagnostic tests such as an ECG
- Diagnostic test results
- Information regarding symptoms and reason for appointment, diagnostic test, or admission
- Physician examinations and record of results, including patient instructions
- Medications and prescriptions given, including refills
- Documentation of informed consent when required
- Legal guardian or representative, if patient is unable to give informed consent

states, "I do not want that electricity going through me!" In a calm manner, you explain that the machine does not produce or generate electricity and it is not harmful. After your explanation, the patient agrees to have the ECG. You have performed successful troubleshooting. Throughout this text, various situations are discussed and potential solutions given. In each chapter, review the "What Should You Do?" questions to check your ability to think critically and troubleshoot.

Troubleshooting **Consent**

When a patient who cannot read or write is required to sign a consent form, you will need to explain the procedure to a family member and have that person sign and the patient sign unless he or she has been determined to be incompetent. If this is not possible, explain the procedure to the patient with a witness present and have the witness sign, along with having the patient place an *X* on the form.

Who should sign the consent form if a patient cannot read or write?

_____

_____

Checkpoint Question 1-5

1. What measures would you use to prevent the spread of infection to you or your patients?

_____

_____

 Answer the preceding question and complete the "What You Need to Know to Perform an ECG" activity on the student CD under Chapter 1 before you proceed to the next section.

Chapter Summary

- An ECG is the tracing of the heart's electrical activity using an electrocardiograph. It is used to diagnose cardiovascular disease which is the number one cause of death in America.
- The heart's electricity was discovered as early as 1676. In 1903, Wilhelm Einthoven is credited developing the first electrocardiograph and introducing the field of electrocardiography.
- Careers in electrocardiography are expanding and include such careers as ECG technician, ECG monitor technician, and cardiovascular technologist.

- The ECG is used routinely in the hospital before surgery, during emergencies, and as part of continuous monitoring. In a clinic an ECG is part of an exam, or used during a treadmill stress test or Holter monitoring. Outside the health care facility, the ECG is used for evaluation during emergencies.
- To perform an ECG you should know the procedure, equipment, and have the ability to communicate and lift and move patients.
- Troubleshooting is the process of critical thinking or thinking through the situation then making a decision to try to solve it. Troubleshooting is a necessary part of performing ECGs.

Chapter Review

Matching

Match these terms with the correct definition. Place the appropriate letter on the line to the left of each term.

_____ **1.** cardiovascular

_____ **2.** electrocardiogram

_____ **3.** arrhythmia

_____ **4.** electrocardiology

_____ **5.** electrocardiograph

_____ **6.** defibrillator

_____ **7.** AED

a. an instrument used to record the electrical activity of the heart

b. a tracing of the signal produced by the heart's electrical activity and used for diagnostic evaluation of the heart

c. the study of the heart's electrical activity

d. abnormal or absence of normal heartbeat, also known as dysrhythmia

e. used to analyze the heart rhythm and produce a shock if necessary

f. related to the heart and blood vessels (veins and arteries)

g. a machine that produces and sends an electrical shock to the heart that is intended to correct the abnormal electrical pattern of the heart

True/False

Read each statement and determine if it is true or false. Circle the T or F. For false (F) statements, correct them to "make them true" on the line provided.

T   F   **8.** An ECG machine produces and records the electrical activity of the heart.

_____   _____

T   F   **9.** Standard precautions are guidelines written for health care providers to help prevent the spread of infection. _____

T   F   **10.** When performing an ECG, you should know the equipment, infection control principles, communication techniques, and safety guidelines. _____

T   F   **11.** A transtelephonic monitor transmits an ECG over the Internet.

_____

Multiple Choice

Circle the correct answer.

12. Which of the following is *not* a reason that an ECG is performed?
   a. To determine how well the heart is pumping
   b. To determine if a person will experience a heart attack in the next month

    c. To check for rhythm abnormalities before surgery

    d. To determine the cause of an irregular heartbeat

13. Which physician invented an instrument to detect electrograph waves?

    a. Sir Thomas Lewis

    b. William Einthoven

    c. Augusta Walker

    d. Joseph Electrocardiograph

14. The first ECG machine was developed in _____ by _____.
   He won the Nobel Prize for this invention.

    a. 1903, Wilhelm Einthoven

    b. 1918, James B. Herrick

    c. 1876, Augusta D. Waller

    d. 1945, Sir Thomas Lewis

15. The main responsibility of an ECG monitor technician is to

    a. Determine whether an abnormal heart rhythm occurs.

    b. View the ECG tracing.

    c. Alert the health care professional.

    d. All of the above.

16. Which of the following is *not* a reason for performing an ECG?

    a. To evaluate heart conditions

    b. To check for problems with the flow of electricity through the heart

    c. To see how well the heart is contracting and pumping

    d. To evaluate the rate and rhythm of breathing

17. A defibrillator can be used

    a. to treat an abnormal heart rhythm.

    b. without training.

    c. to produce an electrical rhythm.

    d. to record only ECG rhythms.

18. Transtelephonic monitoring allows for information to be

    a. reviewed immediately by a physician.

    b. transmitted over a telephone.

    c. submitted for billing purposes only.

    d. recorded by a computerized device.

19. A continuous ECG monitor is used most commonly in a(n)

    a. physician's office.

    b. hospital.

    c. assisted-living center.

    d. clinic.

20. Which of the following is most commonly performed in a clinic or hospital?

    a. Transtelephonic monitoring

    b. Ambulatory monitoring

    c. 12-lead ECG

    d. Defibrillation

21. To write derogatory words about a patient is known as

    a. slander.

    b. libel.

    c. ethical.

    d. unethical.

22. Your most important duties include monitoring an ECG tracing and notifying the physician of abnormalities. You are most likely a(n)
    a. ECG monitor technician.
    b. cardiovascular technologist.
    c. ECG technician or medical assistant.
    d. physician's assistant.

23. Which of the following are measures to ensure that our patients' information is protected?
    a. Standard precautions
    b. Isolation procedures
    c. Patient's bill of rights
    d. HIPAA

24. _____ is the key to successful recording of an ECG.
    a. Hand hygiene
    b. Communication
    c. Patient education
    d. HIPAA

25. What is the single most important procedure you can perform to prevent the spread of infection?
    a. Use of standard precautions
    b. Hand hygiene
    c. Patient education
    d. Communication

26. When speaking to a person who is hard of hearing, it is important that you
    a. Look directly at the patient.
    b. Speak slowly and distinctly.
    c. Speak into the hearing aid if the patient has one.
    d. All of the above.

27. When caring for patients and recording an ECG, you may encounter many situations that require you to
    a. critically think about the situation.
    b. always follow the same steps each time.
    c. not worry about what the patient tells you.
    d. not prepare for what may possibly be asked of you during the procedure.

What Should You Do? *Critical Thinking Application*

Read the following situations and use critical thinking skills to determine how you would handle each. Write your answer in detail in the space provided.

28. You have been performing ECGs at a local clinic for about 6 months. Your favorite uncle says to you, "Since I just turned 40, your Aunt Beth thinks I should have an ECG. Will you do one on me if I come by where you work?" What would you say or do for your uncle? Consider the following:

    Should your uncle have an ECG? _____

    Should you do the ECG if he stops by your office? Why or why not? _____

    _____

    _____

    _____

29. Mr. Smith has been having some mild chest pain. During his ECG, he says, "How does it look? Is there anything wrong?" What would be your best response?

_____

_____

_____

30. You walk by a room where a co-worker is performing an ECG on a female patient. The door is open and the patient is not covered. What would you do?

_____

_____

_____

31. You are responsible for monitoring the heart rhythms on six patients at a local hospital when you begin to feel ill. You are in desperate need to go to the restroom, and you really want to go home. What should you do?

_____

_____

_____

Get Connected *Internet Activity*

Visit the McGraw-Hill Higher Education Online Learning Center *Electrocardiography for Health Care Personnel* Web site at **www.mhhe.com/healthcareskills** to complete the following activity.

History of the ECG If you would like to learn more about the history of the ECG, visit the ECG Library: A brief history of electrocardiography.

Career Exploration If you would like to obtain more information about a career as a cardiovascular technologist or technician, visit the Bureau of Labor Statistics Occupational Outlook Handbook.

Automatic External Defibrillators To learn more about automatic external defibrillators, visit the American Heart Association's Web site and search for the keyword *AED* or *automatic external defibrillator.*

Risk Factors Go to the American Heart Association's Web site. Identify at least five cardiovascular facts related to a specific cultural group and/or identify five risk factors for cardiovascular disease and what can be done to reduce the risk of disease for males or females.

Using the Student CD

Now that your have completed the material in the chapter text, return to the student CD and complete any chapter activities you have not yet done. Practice your terminology with the "Key Term Concentration" game. Review the chapter material with the "Spin the Wheel" game. Take the final chapter test and complete the troubleshooting question and email or print your results to document your proficiency for this chapter.What Is HIPAA?

HIPAA or the Health Insurance Portability and Accountability Act was established in 1996 and passed into law in 2003. It is a national standard for the transfer of health care information. It established security and privacy for exchanging health data electronically and protects patient information. A

The Cardiovascular System

2

Chapter Outline

Learning Outcomes

- Identify the structures of the heart, including valves, chambers, and vessels.
- Compare and contrast pulmonary and systemic circulation.
- Trace the pathway of the blood through pulmonary and systemic circulation.
- Describe coronary circulation.
- Explain the cardiac cycle.
- Identify what takes place during systole and diastole.
- Describe the parts and function of the conduction system.
- Define the unique qualities of the heart and their relationship to the cardiac conduction system.
- Explain the conduction system as it relates to the ECG.
- Discuss the electrical stimulation of the heart as it relates to the ECG waveform.
- Identify each part of the ECG waveform.
- Describe the heart activity that produces the ECG waveform.

Key Terms

aorta	contractility
aortic semilunar valve	coronary circulation
atrioventricular (AV) node	deoxygenated blood
atrium (pl. atria)	depolarization
automaticity	diastole
bundle branches	excitability
bundle of His (AV bundle)	interval
cardiac cycle	interventricular septum
conductivity	ischemia

isoelectric	Purkinje fibers
left atrium	Purkinje network
left ventricle	repolarization
mitral (bicuspid) valve	right atrium
myocardial	right ventricle
oxygenated blood	segment
pericardium	semilunar valve
polarization	sinoatrial (SA) node
pulmonary artery	systemic circulation
pulmonary circulation	systole
pulmonary semilunar valve	tricuspid valve
pulmonary vein	vena cava

2.1 Introduction

The function of the heart is to pump blood to and from all the tissues of the body. Blood supplies the tissues with nutrients and oxygen and removes carbon dioxide and waste products. The process of transporting blood to and from the body tissues is known as circulation. The heart's powerful muscular pump performs the task of circulation. Circulation of the blood is dependent upon the heart and its ability to contract or beat. Each electrical activity of the heart is recorded on the ECG. Knowledge of the heart, its functions, and what produces the ECG tracing will provide you with a clear understanding of the tasks you will be performing as an ECG health care professional.

**Checkpoint
Questions
2-1**

1. What is circulation?

_____

_____

2. What is recorded on the ECG strip?

_____

_____

2.2 Anatomy of the Heart

The heart lies in the center of the chest, under the sternum, and in between the lungs. Two-thirds of it lies to the left of the sternum. It is approximately the size of your fist and weighs about 10.6 ounces or 300 grams (see Figure 2-1).

The heart is a powerful muscular pump that beats an average of 72 times per minute, 100,000 times per day, and 22.5 billion times in the average lifetime. The heart pumps about 140 mL of blood per beat, for a total output of 5 liters per minute. Each day the heart pumps approximately 7250 liters or 1800 gallons of blood. This is enough to fill an average size bathtub about 36 times.

The entire heart is enclosed in a sac of tissue called the **pericardium.** This sac consists of two layers: the tough, outer layer is called the parietal layer, and the inner layer is called the visceral layer. The visceral pericardium adheres closely to the heart. It is also referred to as the epicardium, the outermost layer of the heart. The purpose of the pericardium is to protect

Figure 2-1 The heart is tipped to the left side of the body, and two-thirds of it is located on the left side of the chest.

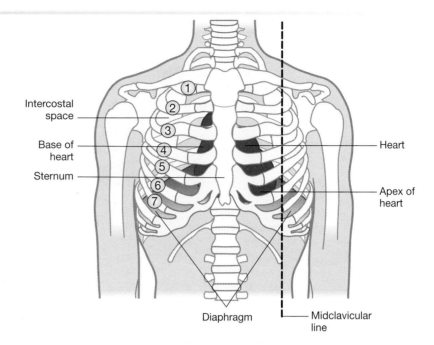

Intercostal space

Base of heart

Sternum

Heart

Apex of heart

Diaphragm

Midclavicular line

the heart from infection and trauma. The space between the two layers is called the pericardial space. It contains about 10 to 20 mL (about ½ ounce) of fluid. This fluid serves to cushion the heart against blows and decreases friction between the layers created by the pumping heart.

The heart consists of three layers: the endocardium, the myocardium, and the epicardium or visceral pericardium. The epicardium, the outermost layer, is thin and contains the coronary arteries. The myocardium is the middle muscular layer that contracts the heart. The endocardium is the innermost layer, which lines the inner surfaces of the heart chambers and the valves. It is also where the Purkinje fibers are located (see Figure 2-2 and Table 2-1).

Chambers and Valves

The heart is divided into four chambers. The top chambers are the **right atrium** and **left atrium.** The bottom chambers are the **right ventricle** and **left ventricle.**

TABLE 2-1 Heart Layers

Layer	Location and Function
Endocardium	Inner layer of the heart that lines the chambers and valves. The Purkinje fibers are located here.
Myocardium	Middle, thickest muscular layer, responsible for heart contraction
Epicardium (also called the visceral pericardium)	Outside, thin layer of the heart that contains the coronary arteries; also the inner layer of the pericardium
Pericardium (made up of the visceral pericardium and the parietal pericardium)	A double-layer sac that encloses the heart. The inner layer, or visceral pericardium, is also called the epicardium; the outer layer is the parietal pericardium.

Figure 2-2 Three distinct layers can be identified on the heart. A sac called the pericardium protects it.

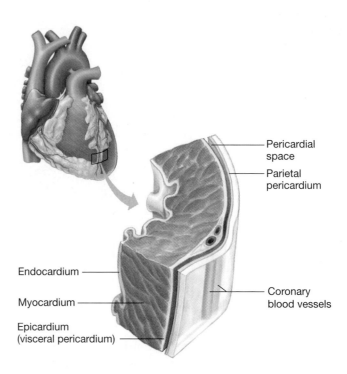

Pericardial space

Parietal pericardium

Endocardium

Myocardium

Epicardium (visceral pericardium)

Coronary blood vessels

Between the right and left ventricle is a partition known as the **interventricular septum.** The myocardium varies in thickness between chambers. It is thin in the atria, thick in the right ventricle, and thickest in the left ventricle. The thicker the myocardium of a chamber is, the stronger the muscular contraction of that chamber. The left ventricle is sometimes known as the "workhorse of the heart" because of its thick myocardium and powerful muscular contraction.

Between the right atrium and right ventricle is the **tricuspid valve.** Between the left atrium and left ventricle is the **mitral (bicuspid) valve.** These two valves are known as atrioventricular valves because they divide the atria from the ventricles. The **pulmonary artery** and the **aorta** each have a **semilunar valve.** They are called semilunar because the valve flaps look like a half (*semi*) moon (*lunar*). These valves are called the **aortic semilunar valve** and the **pulmonary semilunar valve** (see Figure 2-3 and Table 2-2). The semilunar valves separate the ventricles from the arteries leading to the lungs or body.

The one-way valves in the heart keep the blood flow headed in the right direction. The flaps or "cusps" open to allow the blood to flow, then close to prevent the backflow of blood. The mitral (bicuspid) and tricuspid valves

TABLE 2-2 Heart Valves and Their Locations

Name	Valve Type	Location
Aortic	Semilunar	Between left ventricle and aorta
Pulmonary	Semilunar	Between right ventricle and pulmonary artery
Tricuspid	Atrioventricular	Separates right atrium and right ventricle
Mitral (bicuspid)	Atrioventricular	Separates left atrium and left ventricle

Figure 2-3 Heart chambers, valves, and vessels.

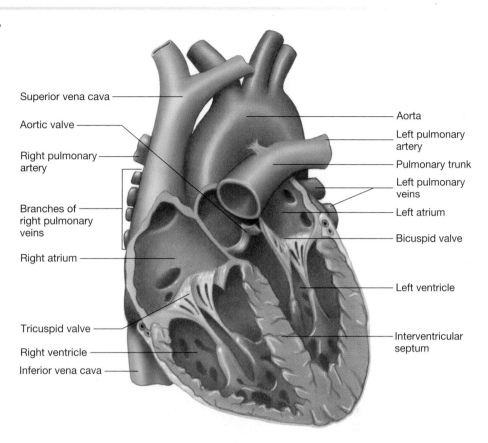

- Superior vena cava
- Aortic valve
- Right pulmonary artery
- Branches of right pulmonary veins
- Right atrium
- Tricuspid valve
- Right ventricle
- Inferior vena cava
- Aorta
- Left pulmonary artery
- Pulmonary trunk
- Left pulmonary veins
- Left atrium
- Bicuspid valve
- Left ventricle
- Interventricular septum

separate the atria and ventricles and prevent the blood from flowing back from the ventricles to the **atria.** The semilunar valves in the pulmonary artery and the aorta prevent the backflow of blood into the ventricles (see Figure 2-4).

The Major Vessels of the Heart

Blood vessels are the veins and arteries that transport blood all over the body. The major blood vessels that transport blood to and from the heart are the vena cava, pulmonary artery, pulmonary veins, and the aorta.

Figure 2-4 Valves viewed from a cross section of the heart.

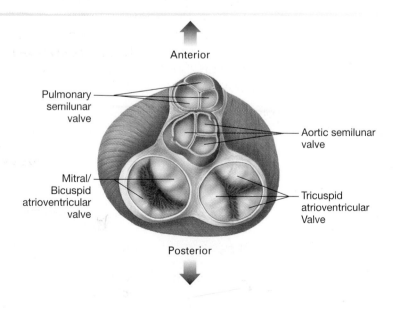

Anterior

- Pulmonary semilunar valve
- Mitral/ Bicuspid atrioventricular valve
- Aortic semilunar valve
- Tricuspid atrioventricular Valve

Posterior

Blood travels from the body tissue through the veins toward the heart. The blood is returned through the largest vein of the body, the **vena cava,** to the right atrium. There are two branches to the vena cava. The superior vena cava transports blood from the head, arms, and upper body. The inferior vena cava transports blood from the lower body and legs.

When the heart contracts, the right ventricle pumps **deoxygenated blood** (blood that has little or minimal oxygen) to the lungs via the pulmonary artery. In the lungs, the exchange of carbon dioxide and oxygen occurs to enrich the blood with oxygen. The **pulmonary veins** transport **oxygenated blood** (blood containing oxygen) back to the heart into the left atrium. Transporting blood to the entire body is the function of the aorta. When the left ventricle contracts, the blood is pumped into the aorta. The first vessels to branch off the aorta are the coronary arteries. Coronary arteries are part of **coronary circulation,** which supplies blood to the muscular heart pump (see Figure 2-5).

Figure 2-5 Pathways for blood through the heart.

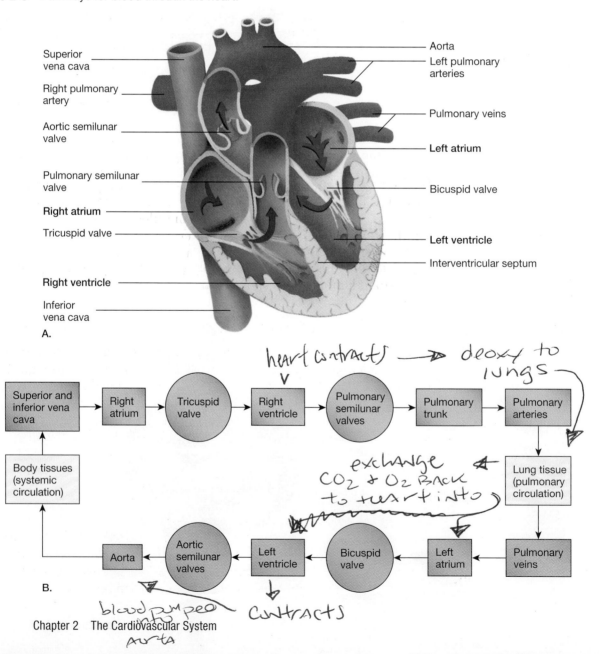

1. What is the middle layer of the heart or the muscular layer?

   _____

   _____

2. What is the valve located between the left atrium and left ventricle?

   _____

   _____

 Answer the preceding questions and complete the "Anatomy of the Heart" activity on the student CD under Chapter 2 before you proceed to the next section.

2.3 Principles of Circulation

The heart is actually a two-sided pump. The left side of the heart pumps oxygenated blood to the body tissue. The right side of the heart pumps deoxygenated blood to the lungs. The pathways for pumping blood to and from the lungs are known as **pulmonary circulation.** The pathways for pumping blood throughout the body and back to the heart are known as **systemic circulation.** The circulation of blood to and from the heart muscle is known as **coronary circulation.**

Pulmonary Circulation: The Heart and Lung Connection

Deoxygenated blood enters the right atrium through the superior and inferior vena cava. Blood travels through the tricuspid valve into the right ventricle. The right ventricle pumps the blood through the pulmonary semilunar valve into the pulmonary artery, then into the lungs. In the lungs, the blood is oxygenated. The blood returns to the heart through the pulmonary veins into the left atrium. The left atrium is the last step of pulmonary circulation.

Systemic Circulation: The Heart and Body Connection

Oxygenated blood enters the left atrium and travels through the mitral valve into the left ventricle. The left ventricle pumps the blood through the aortic semilunar valve into the aorta. The aorta provides the pathway for the blood to circulate through the body. In the body, the oxygen in the blood is exchanged with carbon dioxide. After traveling through the body, the deoxygenated blood returns to the heart through the superior and inferior vena cava (see Figure 2-6).

Coronary Circulation: The Heart's Blood Supply

Oxygenated blood from the left ventricle travels through the aorta to the coronary arteries. There are two main coronary arteries, the left main coronary artery and the right main coronary artery. These arteries branch to supply oxygenated blood to the entire heart. The left main artery has more branches than the right because the left side of the heart is more muscular

Figure 2-6 Pulmonary and systemic circulation.

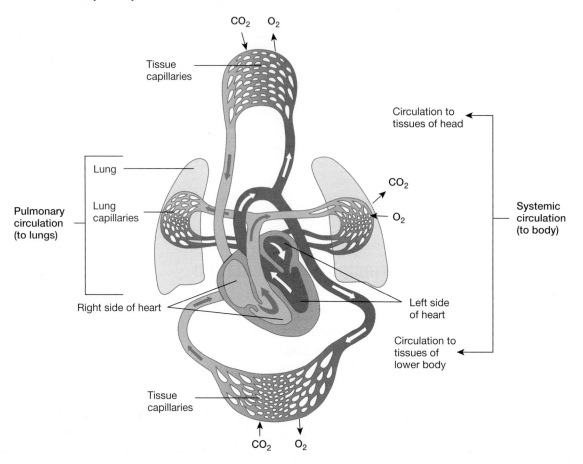

and requires more blood supply. The deoxygenated blood travels through the coronary veins and is collected in the coronary sinus, which empties the blood directly into the right atrium (see Figure 2-7).

Figure 2-7 Coronary circulation.

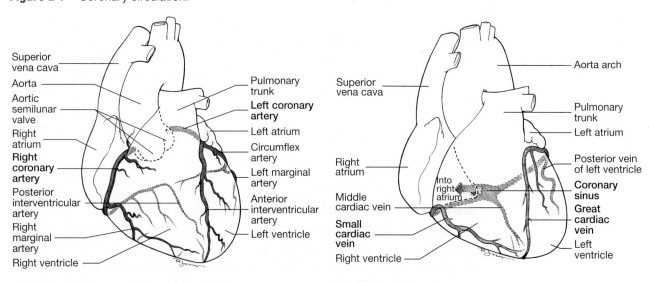

A. Branches of the coronary arteries supply blood to the heart tissue.

B. Branches of the cardiac veins drain blood from the heart tissue.

1. What are the first vessels to branch off the aorta known as?

_____

_____

 Answer the preceding question and complete the "Principles of Circulation" activity on the student CD under Chapter 2 before you proceed to the next section.

2.4 The Cardiac Cycle

Each beat of the heart has two phases that indicate the contraction and the relaxation periods of the heart. The contraction and relaxation of the heart together make up the **cardiac cycle.** When the heart contracts, it is squeezing blood out to the body. As the heart relaxes, it is expanding and refilling. The relaxation phase of the heart is known as **diastole.** The contraction phase is known as **systole.**

Diastole: Relaxation of the Heart

During the diastolic phase, blood from the upper body returns to the heart via the superior vena cava and blood from the lower body returns via the inferior vena cava. The right atrium fills with blood and contracts, pushing open the tricuspid valve. This allows blood to flow into the right ventricle. At the same time, blood is returning from the lungs via the pulmonary veins to the left atrium. This blood fills the left atrium prior to the atrial contraction. The atrial contraction forces the mitral valve open to allow blood to flow into the left ventricle.

Systole: Contraction of the Heart

During the systolic phase, the heart muscle contracts, creating pressure to open the pulmonary and aortic valves. Blood from the right ventricle is pushed into the lungs to exchange oxygen and carbon dioxide. Blood from the left ventricle is pushed through the aorta to be distributed throughout the body to provide oxygen for tissues and remove carbon dioxide.

In adults, the average heart beats approximately 60 to 100 times per minute. In general, women have a faster heartbeat than men. Children's heart rates are usually faster than an adult's heart rate. Children's heart rates depend upon the age and size of the child. If you listen to the heart with a stethoscope, you will hear two sounds: "lubb" and "dupp." These sounds are made by the opening and closing of the heart valves, which is caused by the contraction of the heart. The "lubb" you hear is the sound made during the systolic phase by the contraction of the ventricles and the closing of the mitral and tricuspid valves. The "dupp" sound is made during the diastolic phase. It is shorter and occurs during the beginning of ventricular relaxation. This sound is from the closure of the pulmonary and aortic valves.

Figure 2-8 Diastole and systole.

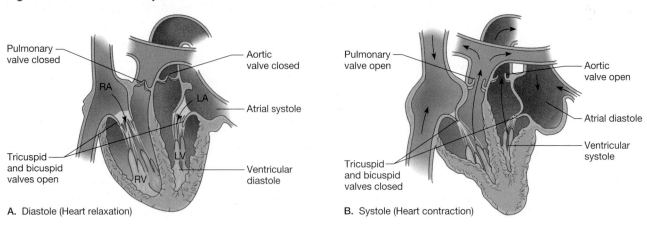

Pulmonary valve closed

Aortic valve closed

RA

LA

Atrial systole

Tricuspid and bicuspid valves open

LV

RV

Ventricular diastole

A. Diastole (Heart relaxation)

Pulmonary valve open

Aortic valve open

Atrial diastole

Ventricular systole

Tricuspid and bicuspid valves closed

B. Systole (Heart contraction)

Each complete "lubb-dupp" you hear is actually one beat of the heart (see Figure 2-8).

Checkpoint Question 2-4

1. What is systole?

_____

_____

Answer the preceding question and complete the "The Cardiac Cycle" activity on the student CD under Chapter 2 before you proceed to the next section.

2.5 Conduction System of the Heart

The pumping cycle or contraction of the heart muscle is controlled by electrical impulses. These impulses are initiated and transmitted through the heart. Specialized masses of tissue in the heart produce these impulses and form the conduction system. The conduction system is necessary for the heart to pump continuously and rhythmically.

Unique Qualities of the Heart

The conduction system is a network of conducting tissue that creates the heartbeat and establishes a pattern for the electrical activity of the heart. The conducting tissue of the heart has several unique qualities. These qualities control the beat of the heart and produce the electrical wave. They include automaticity, conductivity, contractility, and excitability.

Automaticity is the ability of the heart to initiate an electrical impulse without being stimulated by another or independent source. Automaticity is a form of the word *automatic,* which is exactly how the heart beats—automatically. The heart tissue has its own innate ability to initiate an electrical impulse.

The heartbeat relies on the ability of the **myocardial** cells to conduct electrical impulses. (**Myocardial** means pertaining to the heart muscle.) **Conductivity** is the ability of the heart cells to receive and transmit an electrical impulse. The electrical impulse is initiated by automaticity and then travels through the rest of the heart due to the ability of the heart cells to conduct the impulse.

When the heart muscle cells are stimulated by an electrical impulse, they contract. This ability of the heart muscle cells to shorten in response to an electrical stimulus is known as **contractility.** The contraction of the heart muscle cells produces the heartbeat or pumping of the heart.

Excitability is the ability of the heart muscle cells to respond to an impulse or stimulus. Without the quality of excitability, the heart would not react to the electrical impulses that are initiated within the heart.

As you can see, the heart's unique qualities are essential to the rhythmic contraction of the heart muscle and the circulation of blood through the body. Without these qualities, the heart would not beat.

Regulation of the Heart

In addition to automaticity, the heartbeat is controlled by the autonomic nervous system (ANS). Like the unique qualities of the heart, the ANS is involuntary. This means you have no conscious control over its functions. The sympathetic branch of the ANS increases the heart rate by secreting norepinephrine. This happens automatically when you are under stress or become frightened. You can think of the automaticity of the heart as the cruise control in your car. In a normal heart, automaticity sets the rate of the heart to 60 to 100 beats a minute. When the sympathetic branch of the ANS is stimulated, it speeds up the heart. When you let your foot off the accelerator (remove the stimulation to the sympathetic branch of the ANS), the heart rate coasts down to the cruise control speed of 60 to 100.

The parasympathetic branch of the ANS exerts a depressant effect on the heart by secretion of acetylcholine. The vagus nerve is the major nerve of the parasympathetic system and exerts an effect on many of the body organs. It is widespread throughout the body. Stimulation of the vagus nerve slows the heart, acting like a brake to the heart rate. When a patient is experiencing an abnormally fast heart rate, stimulation of the vagus nerve is used to bring the heart back to its normal cruise control rate.

Other factors control the heart. For example, exercise, stress, or a fever can increase the heart rate. Also, the cardiac control center, located in the brain, sends impulses to decrease the heart rate when the blood pressure rises. When the blood pressure falls, it sends impulses to increase the heart rate. The levels of the electrolytes potassium and calcium play a role in the control of the heart. When there is a low concentration of potassium ions in the blood, the heart rate decreases; but a high concentration causes an abnormal heart rate or rhythm. A low concentration of calcium ions in the blood depresses heart actions, but high concentration of calcium causes heart contractions that are longer than normal heart contractions.

Pathways for Conduction

The conduction system consists of the sinoatrial (SA) node, atrioventricular (AV) node, bundle of His (AV bundle), bundle branches, and the Purkinje fibers in the ventricles. The SA and AV nodes are small, round structures that consist of many specialized cardiac cells. The **sinoatrial (SA) node** is located in the upper portion of the right atrium. It is the pacemaker of the heart and initiates the heartbeat. The automaticity of the fibers in the SA node produces the contraction of the right and left atria. The SA node fires at about 60 to100 times per minute. Normal conduction of the heart begins with the SA node.

On the floor of the right atrium is another mass of specialized cardiac cells known as the **atrioventricular (AV) node.** Impulses travel to the AV node because of the unique quality of conductivity through a specialized pathway through the atria. The AV node itself causes a delay (slowdown) in the electrical impulse. This process is important for two reasons. First, it provides time for additional blood to travel from the atria to the ventricles before they contract. This additional blood is known as the atrial kick. The atrial kick increases the cardiac output or the amount of blood that is pumped out of the heart into the body with each contraction. Second, the delay in the electrical impulse reduces the number of electrical impulses transmitted to the ventricles. This is important when the atria are firing too fast. It prevents an excessive rate of electrical impulses from reaching the ventricles. The AV node can also act as the pacemaker if the SA node is not working. It will fire at a rate of 40 to 60 times per minute. This is known as the inherent rate of the AV node.

The **bundle of His (AV bundle),** located next to the AV node, provides the transfer of the electrical impulse from the atria to the ventricles. When the impulse reaches the ventricles, it is divided into the bundle branches. The **bundle branches** are located along the left and right side of the **interventricular septum.** The electrical impulse travels through the right and left bundle branches to the right and left ventricles. The bundle branches are like a fork in the road, and the electrical impulse splits and travels down both sides.

The right and left bundle branches are pathways down the interventricular septum, where the impulses travel to activate the myocardial tissue to contract. Impulses traveling down the left bundle branch will stimulate the interventricular septum to contract in a left-to-right pattern. The ventricles receive their electrical impulses from the bundle branches.

The **Purkinje network** spreads the impulse throughout the ventricles, which occurs through a network of fibers called the **Purkinje fibers.** These fibers provide an electrical pathway for each of the cardiac cells.

Figure 2-9 Conduction pathways.
1. The heartbeat originates in the sinoatrial (SA) node and travels across the wall of the atrium to atrioventricular (AV) node.
2. The impulse passes through the AV node into the AV bundle or Bundles of His to the interventricular septum.
3. The impulse is divided between the right and left bundle branches and travels to the apex of the heart through the interventricular septum via the bundle branches.
4. The Purkinje fibers carry the impulse through the right and left ventricle causing them to contract.

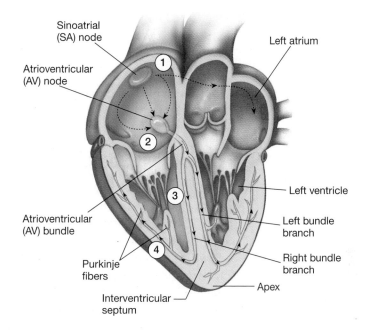

The electrical impulses accelerate and activate the right and left ventricles at the same time to cause the ventricles to contract. The electrical impulse produces an electrical wave (see Figure 2-9 and Table 2-3).

TABLE 2-3   Parts of the Conduction System

Part	Function
Sinoatrial (SA) node (pacemaker)	Initiates heart at a rate of 60 to100 beats per minute with electrical impulse that causes depolarization
Atrioventricular (AV) node	Delays the electrical impulse to allow for the atria to complete their contraction and ventricles to fill before the next contraction
Bundle of His (AV bundle)	Conducts electrical impulses from the atria to the ventricles
Bundle branches	Conducts impulses down both sides of the interventricular septum
Purkinje fibers (network)	Distributes the electrical impulses through the right and left ventricles

1. The ability of the heart muscle cell to respond to a stimulus is called

   _____

   _____

2. Where does the electrical impulse get delayed to allow for all the blood to leave the atrium before the ventricle contracts?

   _____

   _____

 Answer the preceding questions and complete the "Conduction System of the Heart" activity on the student CD under Chapter 2 before you proceed to the next section.

2.6 Electrical Stimulation and the ECG Waveform

Heart cells in their resting state are electrically polarized. This means their insides are negatively charged, whereas on the outside they are positively charged. This state of cellular rest is known as **polarization** and is the ready phase of the heart.

Depolarization, on the other hand, is a state of cellular stimulation, which precedes contraction. It is the electrical activation of the cells of the heart when they lose their internal negativity. Depolarization moves from cell to cell through the electrical pathways. Depolarization is the most important electrical event in the heart—it causes the heart to contract and pump blood to the body.

Repolarization is a state of cellular recovery, which follows each contraction. The cardiac cells return to their resting phase of internal negativity. After depolarization, the cardiac cells return to this state in order to prepare for another depolarization. During repolarization, the heart relaxes and allows for refilling of the chambers of the heart.

The ECG waveform is recorded from the electrical activity produced during depolarization and repolarization of the heart. The waveform on the electrocardiogram is a series of up-and-down deflections off a straight line known as an **isoelectric** line. The isoelectric line represents the period when no electrical activity is occurring in the heart and is known as a baseline. Deflections, which appear as waves on the ECG tracing, indicate electrical activity in the heart. The deflections that go up are positive; the deflections that go down are negative.

When the waveform was first discovered, Einthoven labeled the waves of the electrocardiogram as P, Q, R, S, and T. Legend holds that he chose the letters from the center of the alphabet because he did not know what the waves meant, or whether other waves preceding the P wave or following the T wave would be discovered. The U wave was added after Einthoven's discovery. Each of these waves indicates specific activity in the heart.

In addition to the waves, the ECG waveform contains **intervals, segments,** and complexes. Each of these elements indicates specific activity within the heart. The elements include the QRS complex, the ST segment, the PR interval, and the QT interval (see Table 2-4).

TABLE 2-4 ECG Components

Component	Appearance	Heart Activity
P wave	Upward small curve	Atrial depolarization with resulting atrial contraction
QRS complex	Q, R, and S waves	Ventricular depolarization and resulting ventricular contraction (larger than the P wave); atrial repolarization occurs (not seen)
T wave	Small upward sloping curve	Ventricular repolarization
U wave	Small upward curve	Repolarization of the bundle of His and Purkinje fibers (not always seen)
PR interval	P wave and baseline prior to QRS complex	Beginning of atrial depolarization to the beginning of ventricular depolarization
QT interval	QRS complex, ST segment, and T wave	Period of time from the start of ventricular depolarization to the end of ventricular repolarization
ST segment	End of QRS complex to the beginning of T wave	Time between ventricular depolarization and the beginning of ventricular repolarization

What Each Part of the Waveform Represents

The first deflection is positive and is known as the P wave. This P wave is seen when the atria depolarize. The P wave is small (compared to the other waves of the ECG), rounded, and is the first wave of the normal complex.

During the delay of conduction that occurs at the atrioventricular node, a small baseline segment is seen on the waveform. There is no electrical activity occurring (depolarization or repolarization); thus, no wave or deflection is seen. It is during this time that atrial kick occurs. Atrial kick occurs when the blood is ejected into the ventricles by the atria.

The next three waves occur together as the QRS complex representing ventricular depolarizations. The Q wave represents the conduction of the impulse down the interventricular septum. It is a negative deflection before the R wave. It is not unusual or abnormal for a QRS complex not to have a Q wave. A normal Q wave is less than one fourth of the height of the R wave. The R wave is the first positive wave of the QRS complex. It represents the conduction of electrical impulse to the left ventricle. It is usually the easiest wave to locate on the ECG tracing. The S wave is the first negative deflection after the R wave. It represents the conduction of the electrical impulse through both ventricles. The QRS waves together form the QRS complex. The QRS complex represents ventricular depolarization. It is reflective of the time it takes for the impulses to depolarize the interventricular septum down through the ventricular myocardium causing the ventricles to contract.

The ST segment is measured from the end of the S wave to the beginning of the T wave. This segment should normally be on the isoelectric line. It indicates the end of ventricular depolarization and the beginning of ventricular repolarization. The reason this segment is studied in a 12-lead ECG recording is to determine whether there is any ischemia or myocardial (heart) damage. **Ischemia,** which is lack of blood causing reduced oxygen to the heart muscle, can result in a change in the ST segment. The ST segment will elevate or become depressed depending upon the extent of the ischemia and the amount of damage to the cardiac cells. A change in the ST segment typically indicates some form of injury to the heart muscle. These changes are studied when interpreting an ECG. More information about interpreting an ECG is included in Chapter 5.

The T wave represents ventricular repolarization. As repolarization occurs, the ventricular muscles relax. Normal T waves are in the same direction as the QRS complex and the P wave. A normal T wave peaks toward the end instead of the middle. Unlike the symmetrical mountain shape of the P wave, the T wave looks like a small mountain with one sloping side.

The U wave follows the T wave. The U wave represents repolarization of the bundle of His and Purkinje fibers. The U wave does not always show up on the ECG; however, its presence can indicate an electrolyte imbalance.

The PR interval is measured from the beginning of the P wave to the beginning of the QRS complex. The normal length of time for the PR interval is 0.12 to 0.20 second. The PR interval on a normal ECG should be consistent. This time interval represents the time the electrical impulse is initiated until the ventricles are stimulated by the impulse to start the contraction.

The QT interval is the time required for ventricular depolarization and repolarization to take place. It begins at the beginning of the QRS complex and ends at the end of the T wave. It includes the QRS complex, ST segment, and the T wave.

The R-R interval is the measurement of time from the start of a QRS complex in a rhythm to the start of the next adjacent QRS complex. R waves are readily seen on the ECG and are used to calculate the heart rate in a regular rhythm. We discuss this in Chapter 3.

The junction of the QRS interval and the ST interval is the J point. This represents the end of the QRS complex and ventricular depolarization. The J point is important when measuring the length of the QRS complex and interpreting the ECG tracing. A normal QRS complex is 0.06 to 0.1 second (see Figure 2-10).

Figure 2-10 The ECG waveform and heart activity.

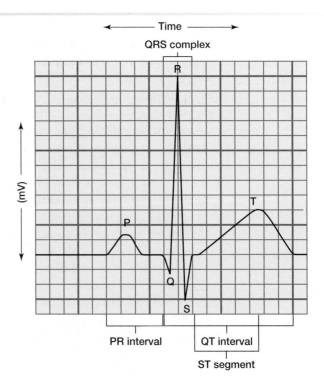

1. Which electrical event is represented by the cardiac contraction of the heart?

   _____

   _____

2. Which wave represents the atrial depolarization?

   _____

   _____

Answer the preceding questions and complete the "Electrical Stimulation and ECG Waveform" activity on the student CD under Chapter 2 before you proceed to the next section.

Chapter Summary

- The heart consists of four chambers (two atria and two ventricles), four major valves (bicuspid, tricuspid and two semilunar valves). The major vessels of the heart include the vena cava, pulmonary artery and veins, and the aorta.
- Pulmonary circulation is transportation of the blood to and from the lungs. Systemic circulation is transportation of blood between the heart and the rest of the body, excluding the lungs.
- Blood travels the following route through the pulmonary and systemic circulation: superior and inferior vena cava—right atrium—tricuspid valve—right ventricle—pulmonary semilunar valve—pulmonary arteries—lungs—pulmonary veins—left atrium—bicuspid valve—left ventricle—aortic valve—aorta—travels through body back to the vena cavas.
- Coronary circulation supplies blood to and from the heart through the coronary arteries and coronary sinus.
- The contraction and relaxation period of the heart together make the cardiac cycle.
- Diastole is the relaxation phase of the cardiac cycle when blood fills the heart. Systole is the contraction phase of the cardiac cycle when blood leaves the heart.
- The conduction system of the heart includes the SA node, AV node, AV bundle, bundle branches, and Purkinje fibers which together create and maintain the electrical activity of the heart.
- The conducting tissue of the conduction system has qualities that control the beat of the heart including automaticity, conductivity, contractility, and excitability.
- The conduction system of the heart creates the electrical activity thus creating the ECG waveform.
- Polarization is the state of cellular rest in the heart. Depolarization is cellular stimulation that causes the heart to contract and repolarization is cellular recovery that follows each contraction.
- The ECG waveform includes the P wave, QRS complex, T wave, U wave (not always seen), PR interval, QT interval, and the ST segment.
- The parts of the ECG waveform are created by the various heart activities of the conduction system including atrial and ventricular depolarization and repolarization.

Chapter Review

Matching

Match the valves, vessels, and chambers of the heart to their definitions. Place the correct letter on the line provided.

_____ 1. left ventricle

_____ 2. tricuspid valve

_____ 3. left atrium

_____ 4. aorta

_____ 5. pulmonary artery

_____ 6. right atrium

_____ 7. right ventricle

_____ 8. semilunar valve

_____ 9. pulmonary vein

_____ 10. mitral valve

a. artery that transports blood to the entire body

b. type of valve located in the aorta and the pulmonary artery

c. atrioventricular valve between the left atrium and left ventricle

d. heart chamber that pumps blood to the body, known as the workhorse of the heart

e. heart chamber that receives blood from the lungs

f. chamber of the heart that receives blood from the body

g. chamber of the heart that pumps blood to the lungs

h. blood vessel that transports blood from the lungs to the left atrium

i. valve located between the right atrium and right ventricle

j. blood vessel that provides a pathway for deoxygenated blood to return to the lungs

Matching II

Match the conduction system parts and unique qualities of the heart to their definitions. Place the correct letter on the line provided.

_____ 11. excitability

_____ 12. automaticity

_____ 13. bundle branches

_____ 14. SA node

_____ 15. contractility

_____ 16. depolarization

_____ 17. AV node

_____ 18. Purkinje fibers

_____ 19. repolarization

_____ 20. conductivity

a. delays the electrical conduction through the heart

b. ability of the heart to initiate an electrical impulse

c. branches off the bundle of His that conduct impulses to the left and right ventricles

d. ability of the heart cells to receive and transmit an electrical impulse

e. an electrical current that initiates the contraction of the heart muscle

f. ability of the heart muscle cells to shorten in response to an electrical stimulus

g. ability of the heart muscle cells to respond to an impulse or stimulus

h. heart muscle cells return to their resting electrical state and the heart muscle relaxes

i. initiates the heartbeat

j. distribute electrical impulses from cell to cell throughout the ventricles

Multiple Choice

Circle the correct answer.

21. The PR interval is usually
    a. 0.06 to 0.10 second.
    b. 0.12 to 0.20 second.
    c. greater than 0.20 second.
    d. less than 0.06 second.

22. What part of the ECG tracing represents the repolarization of the bundle of His and Purkinje fibers?
    a. T wave
    b. PR interval
    c. U wave
    d. P wave

23. What part of the ECG tracing represents the time it takes for the impulse to activate the myocardium to the complete contraction?
    a. WRS complex
    b. J point
    c. QT interval
    d. PR interval

24. What part of the ECG tracing is measured from the end of the S wave to the beginning of the T wave and is normally on the isoelectrial line?
    a. ST segment
    b. QT segment
    c. U wave
    d. QRS complex

25. What wave on the ECG tracing is not always seen and sometimes when seen can indicate an electrolyte imbalance?
    a. U wave
    b. P wave
    c. Q wave
    d R wave

26. The heart's ability to create its own electrical impulse is known as
    a. conductivity.
    b. contractility.
    c. automaticity.
    d. excitability.

27. The sympathetic system of the body causes the heart rate to
    a. increase.
    b. decrease.
    c. remain the same.
    d. none of the above.

28. Which vessel of the body contains the highest concentration of oxygen?
    a. Aorta
    b. Pulmonary artery
    c. Pulmonary vein
    d. Vena cava

29. The heart is contained inside a sac also known as the
    a. endocardium.
    b. pericardial sac.
    c. myocardium sac.
    d. fluid sac.

30. Which of the following would have the *least* effect on the heart rate?
    a. Stress, exercise, and fever
    b. ANS
    c. Potassium and calcium
    d. Respiratory rate

Matching III

Match the information about circulation and the cardiac cycle to the definitions. Place the correct letter on the line provided.

_____ 31. deoxygenated blood

_____ 32. cardiac cycle

_____ 33. systole

_____ 34. coronary circulation

_____ 35. systemic circulation

_____ 36. oxygenated blood

_____ 37. diastole

_____ 38. pulmonary circulation

a. period between the beginning of one beat of the heart to the next
b. circulation of blood through the heart and heart muscle
c. blood that has little or no oxygen
d. phase of the cardiac cycle when the heart is expanding and refilling; also known as the relaxation phase
e. blood having oxygen
f. circulation between the heart and the entire body, excluding the lungs
g. transportation of blood to and from the lungs
h. contraction phase of the cardiac cycle, when the heart is pumping blood out to the body

Label the Parts

39. a.–o. Label the vessels, valves, and chambers of the heart by using the letters of the terms.

   a. Right atrium
   b. Aorta
   c. Right ventricle
   d. Right pulmonary veins
   e. Left atrium
   f. Left ventricle
   g. Superior vena cava
   h. Pulmonary trunk
   i. Aortic valve
   j. Tricuspid valve
   k. Right pulmonary artery
   l. Mitral (bicuspid) valve
  m. Inferior vena cava
   n. Left pulmonary veins
   o. Left pulmonary artery
   p. Interventricular septum

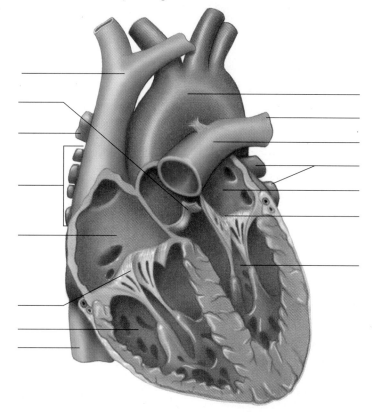

40. a.–n. Label the following diagram representing the flow of blood through the heart. Write the letters of the terms in the appropriate circle or box.

   a. Superior and inferior vena cava
   b. Right atrium
   c. Aorta
   d. Right ventricle
   e. Pulmonary semilunar valves
   f. Left atrium
   g. Bicuspid valve

   h. Pulmonary trunk
   i. Pulmonary veins
   j. Tricuspid valve
   k. Left ventricle
   l. Aortic semilunar valve
  m. Pulmonary arteries

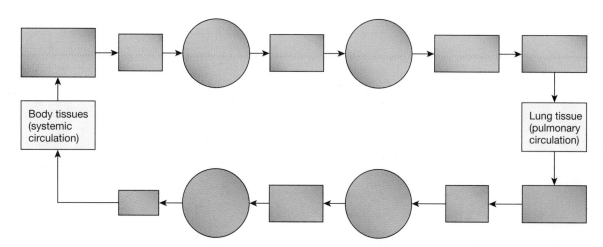

41. a.–h. Label the parts of the conduction system. Write the letter on the lines provided.

   a. Interventricular septum
   b. Left bundle branch
   c. Purkinje fibers
   d. AV node
   e. SA node
   f. AV bundle
   g. Right bundle branch
   h. Apex

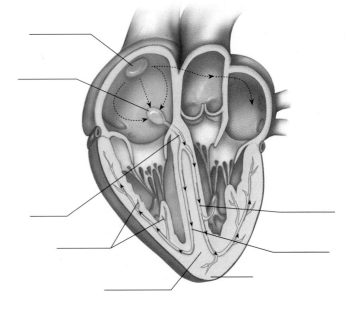

42. a.–i. Label the waves, complexes, intervals, and segments of the ECG waveform. Write the letter of the terms in the appropriate box.

   a. S wave
   b. R wave
   c. P wave
   d. T wave
   e. Q wave
   f. QT interval
   g. ST segment
   h. QRS complex
   i. PR interval

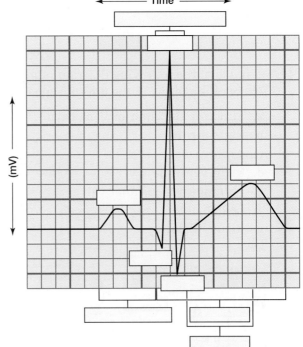

Right or Wrong?

43. You and a friend have just finished studying this chapter. Your friend makes the following statements. Are his or her statements correct or incorrect? If the statement is incorrect, write down what you would say to correct your friend.

a. "The valves between the atria and the ventricles are semilunar." _____

_____

b. "The atria always pump the blood." _____

_____

c. "The heart is a two-sided pump that produces pulmonary circulation and systemic circulation."_____

_____

d. "The coronary arteries carry deoxygenated blood." _____

_____

e. "The pulmonary artery carries oxygenated blood." _____

_____

f. "The waves on the ECG waveform are positive when they are up and negative when they are down."_____

_____

g. "If you are a man, you will have a faster heartbeat." _____

_____

h. "The top chambers of the heart are the ventricles, and the bottom chambers of the heart are the atria." _____

_____

i. "The right ventricle is sometimes known as the workhorse of the heart." _____

_____

j "The waves of the ECG waveform are P, Q, R, S, T, and sometimes a U." _____

_____

Voyage Through the Heart

44. For each of the following statements, identify the vessel or structure you are in. Write in the space provided. Imagine you are a drop of blood traveling through the heart. Returning from the brain, you are about ready to enter the heart.

   a. What vessel are you in? _____

   _____

   b. After you enter the right atrium, you have to go through a door in order to enter the right ventricle. What is the name of this door? _____

   _____

   c. You have made it to the lungs successfully and are traveling back to the heart. What vessels are you in? _____

   _____

   d. When you get to the heart, where will you be? _____

   _____

   e. You have finally made it to the last chamber of the heart. The left ventricle pumps you into the entire body. After entering the aorta, what are the very first vessels you will travel into?

   _____

What Should You Do? *Critical Thinking Application*

Read the following situations and use your critical thinking skills to determine how you would handle each. Write your answer in detail in the space provided.

45. When the atria outside of the SA node stimulates the atria to beat too fast, this is known as atrial flutter or atrial fibrillation. When these heart rhythms occur, the ventricles do not beat at the same rate as the atria. What part of the conduction system prevents the ventricles from beating as fast as the atria and how does it occur?

   _____

   _____

46. You are working in the emergency room recording an ECG when the electricity goes out. There is a short period of darkness followed by a very loud noise. When you regain power, the hearts of both you and your patient are beating extremely fast. What part of the cardiovascular system is responsible for this increased heart rate? Should you continue recording the ECG now or later, and why?

   _____

   _____

Get Connected *Internet Activity*

Visit the McGraw-Hill Higher Education Online Learning Center *Electrocardiography for Health Care Personnel* Web site at **www.mhhe.com/healthcareskills** to complete the following activity.

Visit the National Heart, Lung, and Blood Institute's Web site for Web link for OLC information about coronary heart disease. Create a patient education brochure called, "How to Prevent Coronary Heart Disease" from what you learn.

Visit the Web site "Get Body Smart" and review information about the heart to prepare for the chapter test.

Using the Student CD

Now that you have completed the material in the chapter text, return to the student CD and complete any chapter activities you have not yet done. Practice your terminology with the "Key Term Concentration" game. Review the chapter material with the "Spin the Wheel" game. Take the final chapter test and complete the troubleshooting question and email or print your results to document your proficiency for this chapter.

3 The Electrocardiograph

Learning Outcomes

- Identify the three types of leads.
- Explain how each lead is recorded.
- Compare and contrast the differences between a single channel and a multichannel ECG machine.
- List the functions of common ECG machines.
- Discuss the ECG machine controls and identify how each control is used.
- Describe the parts of the electrocardiograph.
- Identify common electrodes.
- Describe the ECG graph paper.
- Identify the measurements of an ECG waveform on the ECG graph paper.

Key Terms

artifact
augmented
bipolar
bradycardia
Einthoven triangle
electrodes
gain
input
lead
limb
mm (millimeter)

multichannel recorder
mV (millivolt)
output display
precordial
signal processing
single-channel recorder
speed
standardization
stylus
tachycardia
unipolar

3.1 Introduction

In Chapter 2, you learned about the heart's conduction system and how the ECG waveform is produced. In this chapter, we discuss the electrocardiograph and the equipment needed to perform an ECG and record the ECG waveform. You will discover how the 12-lead system works and what the measurements are on the ECG graph paper. Learning the equipment and lead system thoroughly and correctly will prepare you to record your first ECG.

Checkpoint Question 3-1

1. What will you need to know to prepare yourself for recording your first ECG?

_____

_____

3.2 Producing the ECG Waveform

The electrical impulse that is produced by the heart's conduction system is measured with the ECG machine. The ECG machine interprets the impulse and produces the ECG waveform. The waveform indicates how the heart is functioning electrically. Since the heart is three dimensional, it is necessary to view the electrical impulse and heart functioning from different sides. A single heart rhythm tracing views the heart from one angle. A 12-lead ECG is a complete picture of the heart's electrical activity, looking at it from 12 different angles as you might look at a sculpture. It records the heart's electrical activity in 12 different views at slightly different angles. The 12-lead ECG records the electrical impulses produced in the heart. It is not a picture of the heart structure; it is a recording of the electrical activity within the heart. The 12 views provide information about how the electrical impulses travel through various parts of the heart.

A 12-lead ECG is actually recorded by only 10 lead wires, which, when attached to the chest and the **limbs** (arms and legs), provide the 12 different views for the 12-lead tracing. Six of these leads attach to the chest electrodes, and the other four attach to the electrodes on the arms and legs or shoulders and lower abdomen. **Electrodes** are small sensors placed on the skin to receive the electrical activity from the heart, and **leads** are covered wires that conduct the electrical impulse from the electrodes to the ECG machine. The lead wires are identified by color and are labeled with letters to match the correct position on the patient's body (see Table 3-1 and Figure 3-1).

TABLE 3-1 Lead Identification

Identifying Letters	Designated Color	Lead Wire Placement
RA	White	Right arm
LA	Black	Left arm
RL	Green	Right leg
LL	Red	Left leg
V1–V6	Brown	Chest leads

Troubleshooting

Check the Lead Wires

Each of the lead wires is coded by color and letter. If you place the lead wires incorrectly, the ECG will not record at all or it will record the waveforms improperly. Always check and double-check the lead wires before you begin the tracing. An ECG recording produced with the lead wires attached incorrectly is not acceptable and will have to be repeated.

If you attempt to record an ECG and no tracing is seen, what should you do?

_____

_____

Figure 3-1 When attaching the lead wires, check carefully for the correct color- and letter-coded wire.

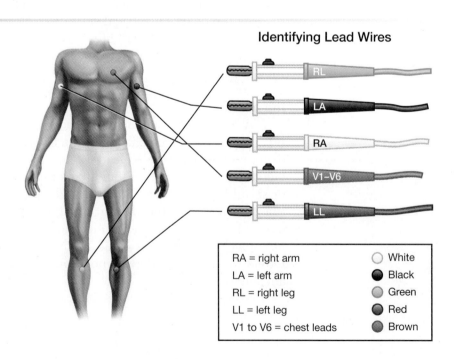

Identifying Lead Wires

RA = right arm — ○ White
LA = left arm — ● Black
RL = right leg — ○ Green
LL = left leg — ● Red
V1 to V6 = chest leads — ● Brown

The 10 lead wires produce 12 different lead circuits consisting of one or more wires from the electrodes to the electrocardiograph. The 12 circuits produce 12 different tracings or views of the heart. The electrodes, or a combination of electrodes, identify each of the 12 leads. The 12 leads are made up of three different types of leads: three standard limb leads, three augmented leads, and six chest leads.

To understand the circuits for the first six leads (three standard and three augmented) we can use the Einthoven triangle. Einthoven is the scientist credited with developing the first ECG machine. The **Einthoven triangle** is formed by three of the limb electrodes: those on the right arm, the left arm, and the left leg. The right leg is used only as a ground or reference electrode (see Figure 3-2).

The electrical current created by the heart is measured between the positive and negative electrodes placed on the body. If no current is flowing, the waveform is flat, or isoelectric. If the current moves toward the positive electrode, the ECG waveform will be positive, or upright, above the isoelectric baseline. If the current moves away from the positive electrode or toward the negative electrode, the ECG waveform will be negative, or downward, below the isoelectric baseline.

Standard Limb Leads

The first three leads are known as standard limb leads. They are also known as **bipolar** leads because they measure the flow of electrical current in two directions at the same time. These first three leads are called lead I, lead II, and lead III. In the Einthoven triangle, leads I, II, and III are positioned at the same distance from the heart's electrical activity. Lead I records the tracing from the right arm (−) to the left arm (+) and produces a positive wave. Lead II records the tracing from the right arm (−) to the left leg (+) and produces a positive or upward deflection. Lead III records the electrical activity traveling from the left arm (−) to the left leg (+) (see Figure 3-3).

Augmented Leads

The second three leads are known as **augmented** leads because their tracings are increased in size by the ECG machine in order to be interpreted. They are also known as **unipolar** leads because they measure toward one electrode

Figure 3-2 The Einthoven triangle helps us understand the reference points for the 12-lead ECG.

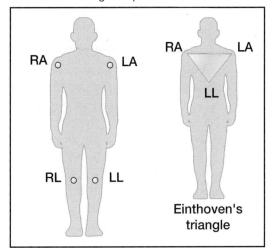

Einthoven's triangle

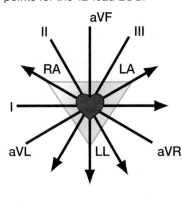

Figure 3-3 Leads I, II, and III are standard limb leads and are recorded from these reference points on the Einthoven triangle producing a positive deflection.

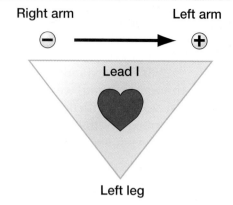

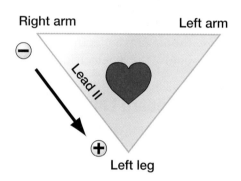

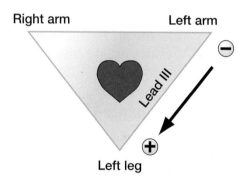

on the body. They are called aVR, aVL, and aVF. The R, L, and F refer to the direction the lead is measuring: R is right arm, L is left arm, and F is foot (see Figure 3-4). Lead aVR records electrical activity from midway between the left arm and left leg to the right arm. Lead aVR is usually a negative deflection. If it does not produce a negative deflection, you might have the electrodes or lead wires placed incorrectly. To ensure accuracy of electrodes and lead wire placement, check the aVR tracing produced when recording the 12-lead ECG; if it is not a negative deflection, verify the placement of the electrodes and lead wires to correct it.

Lead aVL records electrical activity from the midpoint between the right arm and left leg to the left arm. Lead aVF records electrical activity from the midpoint between the right arm and left arm to the left leg. The voltage is very low with the augmented leads because of the angle of measurement; therefore, the ECG waveform will be very small. The ECG machine must increase (augment) the size of the waveforms for these leads to be readable on the ECG tracing.

Figure 3-4 The augmented leads aVR, aVL, and aVF are recorded from midway between two points on the Einthoven triangle. Because of the lead reference points, their tracings are normally small but are augmented (enlarged) by the ECG machine.

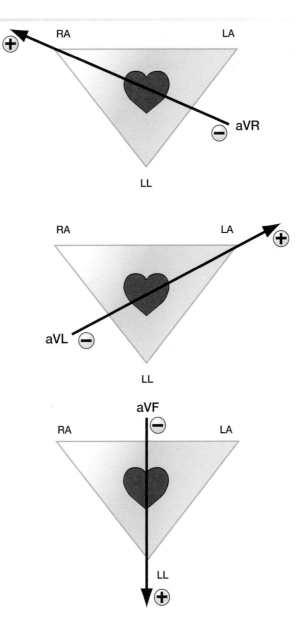

Chest Leads

The last six leads are the chest leads. Also known as **precordial,** these leads are located in front of (*pre*) the heart (*cor*). The chest leads are unipolar because they are measured in one direction only. They are placed on specific sites on the chest. Each of the chest leads begins with the letter V and is numbered from V1 to V6. These leads record activity between six points on the chest and within the heart. You can view the placements in Figure 3-5. The procedure for placing electrodes is discussed in Chapter 4, "Performing an ECG."

The 12-lead ECG tracings can be interpreted separately or in conjunction with each other. When an ECG is being recorded, each of the 12 leads must be identified on the tracing. Older machines required that the ECG tracing strip be coded with identifying marks manually. Most machines identify each lead tracing automatically. Each lead tracing looks slightly different and presents a different picture of the heart. This allows the physician to determine damage or problems in specific areas of the heart (see Figure 3-6).

Figure 3-5 Front and cross section view of chest lead placement.

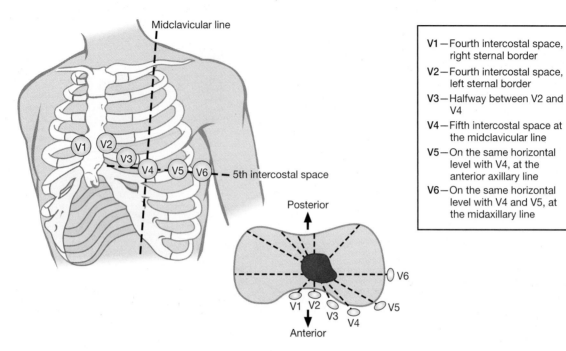

Midclavicular line

V1 — Fourth intercostal space, right sternal border

V2 — Fourth intercostal space, left sternal border

V3 — Halfway between V2 and V4

V4 — Fifth intercostal space at the midclavicular line

V5 — On the same horizontal level with V4, at the anterior axillary line

V6 — On the same horizontal level with V4 and V5, at the midaxillary line

5th intercostal space

Posterior

Anterior

Figure 3-6 A 12-lead ECG produced on a multichannel ECG machine. Each lead is identified on the printout. Note the difference in appearance of the tracings from the 12 leads.

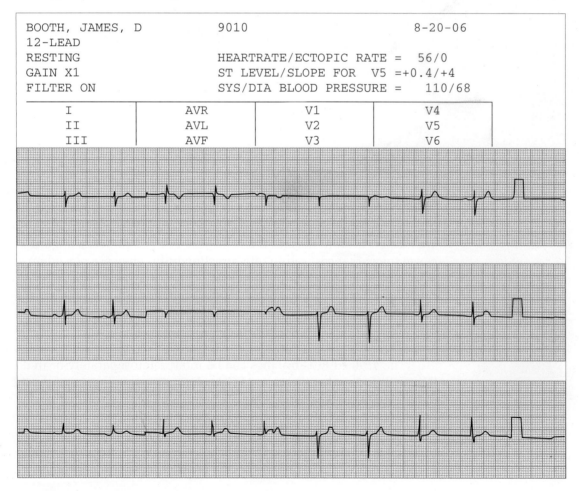

```
BOOTH, JAMES, D          9010                    8-20-06
12-LEAD
RESTING              HEARTRATE/ECTOPIC RATE =  56/0
GAIN X1              ST LEVEL/SLOPE FOR  V5 =+0.4/+4
FILTER ON           SYS/DIA BLOOD PRESSURE =   110/68

        I           AVR           V1            V4
        II          AVL           V2            V5
        III         AVF           V3            V6
```

Figure 3-7 A 15-lead tracing is an expanded view of the heart and may include a specific focus on the right ventricle or posterior of the heart. V3R, V4R, and V8 are additional tracings that are recorded in addition to the first 12 leads.

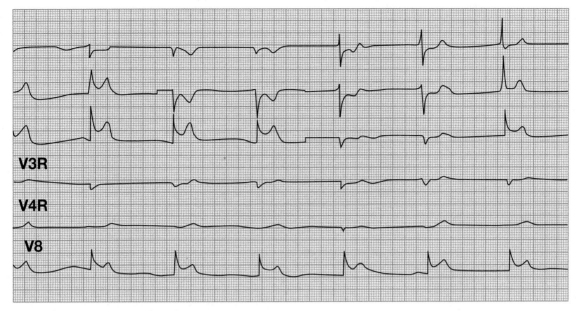

In some situations, the chest leads may be expanded to view all sides of the heart. These 15-lead or more views may include specific focus on the right ventricle or posterior (backside) of the heart (see Figure 3-7).

Checkpoint Questions 3-2

1. How many lead wires are used to obtain a 12-lead ECG tracing?

   _____

   _____

2. Name three augmented leads

   _____

   _____

 Answer the preceding questions and complete the "Producing the ECG Waveform" activity on the student CD under Chapter 3 before you proceed to the next section.

3.3 ECG Machines

Machines used today to measure an ECG weigh less than 10 pounds; some are as small as a credit card. All ECG machines vary slightly, but most have the same basic parts. The typical ECG machine sits on a small cart that can be pushed to the person requiring the ECG. You should become familiar with the type of machine you will be using by reading the manufacturer's instructions.

Types of ECG Machines

There are two main types of ECG machine recorders: single-channel recorders and multichannel recorders. The **single-channel recorder** monitors 12 leads individually; it produces a strip 3 to 6 feet long showing all 12 leads (see Figure 3-8). The recorded ECG tracing strip may need to be cut and mounted,

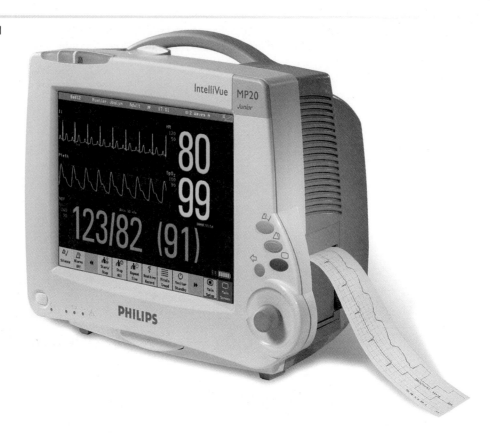

Figure 3-8 A single-channel ECG machine records only one lead at a time and uses a roll of paper that produces a single lead strip.

or placed on a card, for interpretation. Each lead is marked on the strip while the ECG is recording. The ECG tracing must be mounted correctly to ensure proper interpretation by the physician. Read the directions carefully and place each lead tracing in the correct location. Mounting a single-channel ECG tracing is discussed in more detail in Chapter 4.

The **multichannel,** three-channel ECG **recorder** monitors all 12 leads but records three leads at once and switches automatically, recording each of the four sets of three leads. As seen in Figure 3-6, it produces a full sheet of paper showing all 12 lead tracings. The actual recording time for this machine is approximately 10 seconds (see Figure 3-9). This tracing does not usually need to be mounted, but it may need to be attached to a thicker backing or copied when filed permanently with the health care provider's interpretation. Also available are multichannel ECG machines that can record up to six lead tracings at one time. As technology advances, electronic copies of 12-lead tracings and interpretations are being stored and transmitted electronically via telecommunications.

Functions

There are three basic functions of the electrocardiograph: input, signal processing, and output display. Sensors in the ECG machine serve as receiving devices for the electrical activity of the heart. Electrodes placed on the patient's skin direct the impulses to the ECG instrument, providing the **input** for the ECG machine.

Signal processing occurs inside the ECG machine. It amplifies the electrical impulse and converts it into mechanical actions on the display. A complex collection of transistors, resistors, and circuitry amplify and prepare the signal for transfer to the output display.

Figure 3-9 A multichannel ECG machine records 3, 4, or 6 leads at a time on a large sheet of ECG graph paper.

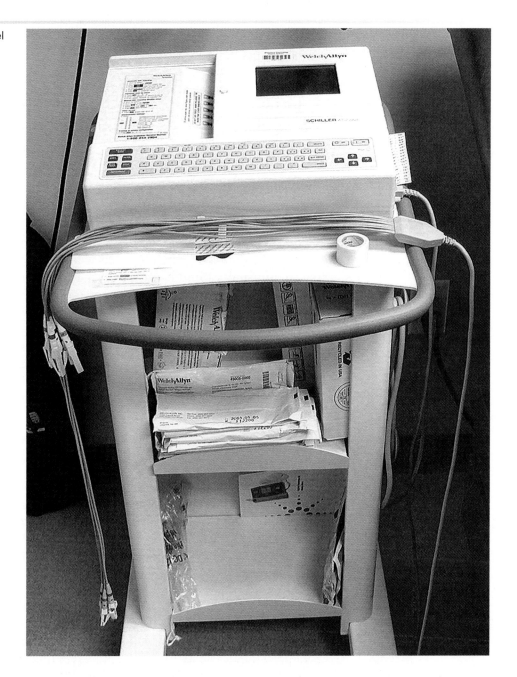

The **output display** is the result of the ECG tracing. Commonly, this is the printed report or computerized data report. The output can also appear on a screen known as an oscilloscope. An oscilloscope is frequently found on a cardiac monitor or a defibrillator. For a 12-lead ECG, the printed format is an important output display since it provides a hard copy of the information.

ECG machines also perform other functions as well, including computerized measurement and analysis, storage, and communication. Computerized measurement and analysis provide a machine interpretation of the ECG. This interpretation is not meant to replace the physician's interpretation. However, the computer interpretation can distinguish between a normal and abnormal recording quickly and may provide a second opinion. All computerized interpretation needs to be validated by a physician.

Some ECG machines store ECG results, which can be recalled and printed later. ECG machines are also equipped to transmit results over the telephone, fax, or Internet. As technology is being improved, you should stay current on the latest changes and advancements to the equipment you will be using.

Controls

The three most important controls on the electrocardiograph include the speed, gain, and artifact filter.

Speed

The **speed** control regulates how fast or slow the paper or data run during the ECG procedure. The most commonly used standard rate is 25 millimeters per second (written as 25 **mm**/sec). In some cases, you may want to increase the speed to 50 mm/sec, which is twice as fast. You would do this if the patient has an unusually rapid heart rate. It may also be done if the ECG waveform parts are too close together. Increasing the speed would allow the waveform to be analyzed more easily. Some ECG machines allow you to reduce the speed to 5 mm/sec or 10 mm/sec in order to analyze the ECG recording more carefully. Changing the speed of the recorder is usually done at the request or preference of the physician. Remember, if you change the speed to anything other than the standard 25 mm/sec, you must note this on the tracing and notify the health care provider who will interpret the tracing, if possible.

Troubleshooting **Changing the ECG Tracing Speed**

When the patient's heart rate is very fast, it will be difficult to read the ECG tracing because the waveform parts will be close together. Set the speed control at 50 mm/sec to widen the complexes so the ECG can be interpreted more easily. Circle or note the speed setting and, when possible, verbally tell the health care provider who will be interpreting the results the change in speed. A normal ECG set to double speed can sometimes look like an abnormal rhythm known as a heart block.

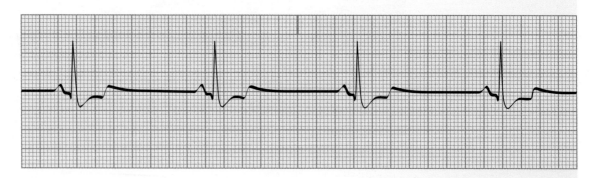

This ECG tracing was produced at a speed of 50 mm/sec. What should you do?

_____

_____

Know Your ECG Machine

Become familiar with the ECG machine you will be using before performing an ECG. Your uncertainty could cause anxiety or nervousness in the patient who is having the ECG performed.

Gain

The **gain** control regulates the output or height of the ECG waveform. The normal setting is 10 mm/**mV** (millivolts are the units of measurement used to indicate voltage on the ECG tracing). By setting the gain to 20 mm/mV, you can double the size; by setting the gain to 5 mm/mV, you reduce the size by half. Some machines will let you change the gain depending on which lead you are tracing. Since the tracing size can vary between leads, setting the gain will allow the ECG waveform to be readable for any lead tracing. If you change the gain setting during any lead tracing, you must record this change on the ECG report.

Artifact Filter

The ECG machine you are using may have an **artifact** filter selection. The usual setting is between 40 Hz (hertz, a unit of frequency that indicates per second) and 150 Hz. Forty Hz is normally used to reduce artifact or abnormal marks on the ECG tracing due to muscle tremor and slight patient movement. We discuss artifact in more detail in Chapter 4. Remember that the artifact filter will correct only the printed output. If the computer performs interpretation, it will interpret the results from the actual nonfiltered information from the patient, not what is printed or viewed on the screen. This could cause inaccurate interpretation by the computer, which is why it is essential that a physician as well as the computer interpret all ECGs. Some filtering of artifact will prohibit the view of pacemaker spikes. It is important to know how to modify the filter to allow for pacemaker spikes to be seen.

LCD Display

There are various other controls on the ECG machine that the user can set or use to enter information. For example, the user can enter data about the patient to be included on the printout along with the ECG results. This information would be entered into the LCD (liquid crystal diode) display (see Figure 3-10). This is the area of the machine where you can view the patient information you have entered. It is also where information from the ECG's computer is displayed. For example, a newer machine can detect if the arm leads or chest leads are reversed, and it will display this information in the LCD panel.

Heart Rate Limits

If the ECG machine has computer interpretation, the user may be able to set the heart rate limits. In other words, the operator can set the heart rate that the machine will interpret as too slow—**bradycardia**—or too fast—**tachycardia.** If the heart rate is above or below the number set, the machine will indicate this by sounding an alarm and marking on the tracing.

Figure 3-10 On many ECG machines, information is entered into the LCD display. Some machines can even identify incorrect lead placement.

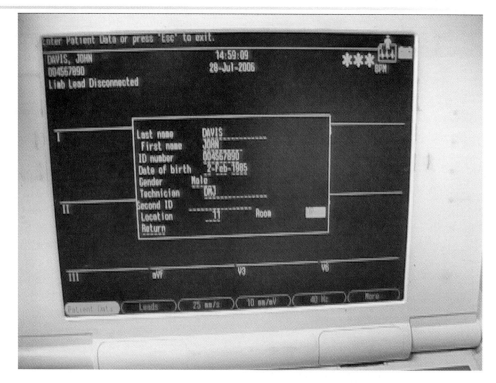

Troubleshooting

Changing the Gain

When the deflections on the ECG tracing are too short or tall, you will need to correct the gain. Be certain the machine is standardized correctly and then adjust the gain control if necessary.

When recording an ECG and the deflections or spikes of the tracing are not large enough, what should you do?

_____

_____

Stylus and Standardization Control

Older ECG machines write on special paper with a heated **stylus.** The stylus reacts with the treated paper and produces a tracing. When the heat is turned up, a darker tracing results; when the heat is turned down, it produces a light tracing. The heat should be set so the tracing is clear and not too dark to avoid smearing or bleeding. Machines with a stylus must be standardized before use.

If you are using a machine that requires **standardization,** this procedure must be done in order to ensure that the machine is recording correctly. Pressing the standardization control produces a standardization mark. The stylus should move up 10 small squares and remain there for two small squares. If this does not occur, the machine must be adjusted before use. To make this adjustment, check the manufacturer's directions for the machine you are using.

Newer digital machines use thermal technology, which is achieved by heating dots as the paper moves across the print head. Digital machines

Figure 3-11 The calibration mark on the ECG tracing must be verified to ensure accuracy. The first square waveform on the ECG tracing is indicating the standardization of the machine for the recorded ECG.

Calibration marks

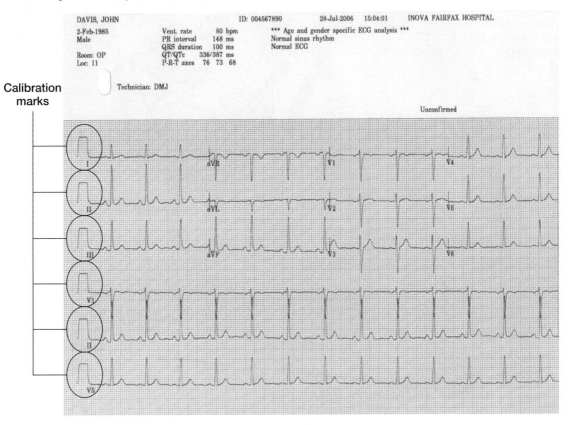

require no manual standardization; the machine makes the adjustments automatically. However, a calibration or standardization mark must be seen on the tracing (see Figure 3-11).

Lead Selector

Most 12-lead ECG machines record each of the leads automatically. However, a lead selector is used to run each lead individually in case one or more leads needs to be repeated.

Checkpoint Questions 3-3

1. A multichannel ECG monitors all 12 leads but usually records how many leads at one time?

   _____

   _____

2. What are some reasons that you may change the speed of the ECG tracing?

   _____

   _____

 Answer the preceding questions and complete the "ECG Machines" activity on the student CD under Chapter 3 before you proceed to the next section.

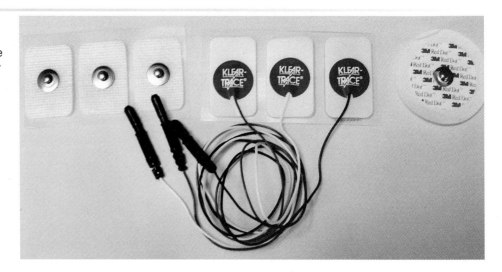

Figure 3-12 Disposable electrodes come in various shapes and sizes. Electrolyte gel or paste is not necessary since it is already contained on these electrodes.

3.4 Electrodes

Electrodes are sensors that are placed on a person's skin to pick up the electrical activity of the heart and conduct it to the ECG machine. The standard 12-lead ECG uses 10 electrodes. These electrodes come in a variety of types and are usually disposable. Reusable electrodes are essentially a thing of the past. If used, they however, do require care and maintenance.

Disposable Electrodes

Disposable electrodes are used because they reduce the possibility of cross-contamination and can be simply removed and discarded for easier cleanup (see Figure 3-12). The self-adhesive types stick easily to the patient's body. The gel is already applied so the electrodes will properly conduct the electrical impulses.

Safety and Infection Control

Do Not Mix Electrodes

You should never mix two different types of electrodes. This could cause an inaccurate tracing, which could result in incorrect treatment for the patient.

Each disposable electrode is normally used on only one ECG. The only exception occurs when a second ECG is performed on the same patient immediately after the first and the electrodes are not disturbed. For example, if you are transferring a patient from an outpatient facility to a hospital, you should leave the electrodes in place for the emergency medical personnel. They will be recording one or more ECGs on the way to the hospital. If the electrodes stay on the patient's skin any longer than two sequential readings, the gel will dry out, resulting in inaccurate ECG tracings.

For hospitalized patients, longer-lasting silver electrodes are available. These electrodes are used for patients who require multiple and frequent ECGs (serial ECGs). When serial ECGs are required, it is important to ensure the same lead placement for each. A slight change often causes a change in the tracing. The silver electrodes are kept on the patient and checked daily.

No matter what type of electrodes are used, they must be handled and stored correctly. If a package contains more electrodes than needed, the remaining electrodes must be kept in a sealed plastic bag so the gel will not dry out. Always check the expiration date on the package before use. Make sure the electrode gel has not dried out on any electrode. Even new electrodes should be checked before placement.

Checkpoint Question 3-4

1. Which type of electrode is used when monitoring a patient that will be having serial ECGs done?

_____

_____

 Answer the preceding question and complete the "Electrodes" activity on the student CD under Chapter 3 before you proceed to the next section.

3.5 ECG Graph Paper

The ECG machine records an image of the heart's electrical activity onto graph paper. This image is the ECG waveform, or a series of waves and complexes recorded from the activity in the heart. The graph paper provides increments to measure the electrical activity produced on the tracing. Understanding the ECG paper is a necessary part of performing an ECG and is essential to interpreting the ECG (see Figure 3-13).

The two most commonly used types of paper are standard grid and dot matrix. Both are heat and pressure sensitive. Because the paper is pressure

Figure 3-13 Choose the right size and type of graph paper for the ECG machine you will be using.

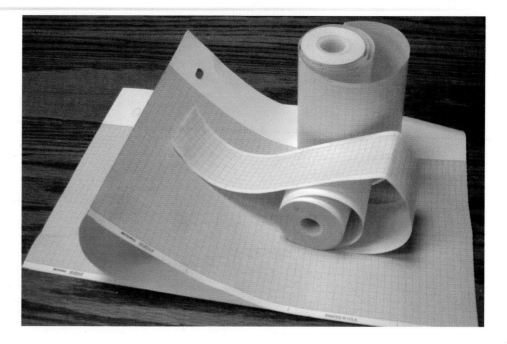

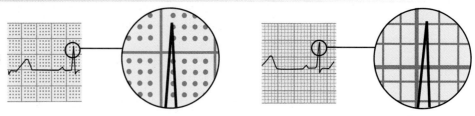

Figure 3-14 Comparison of ECG graph paper: dot matrix paper (left) requires less ink, is easier to read, and produces sharper photocopies, whereas standard grid paper (right) is slightly less expensive.

sensitive, you should handle it carefully to avoid marking it. Marks on the paper could make the tracing difficult to read or inaccurate. In addition, certain substances such as alcohol, plastic, sunlight, and X-ray film can erase the tracing. Once the ECG is completed, it should be stored away from these substances. Some companies offer recording paper that requires no special handling or storage. This paper guarantees that the tracing will last for up to 50 years.

Troubleshooting **Handle the ECG Report with Care**

Handle and store the ECG report with care. It can be damaged easily; and, if damaged, it cannot be interpreted by the physician.

The physician places a stack of charts on top of an ECG report you just placed on his desk. What should you do?

_____

_____

Dot matrix paper has some advantages over standard grid paper. Dot matrix reports require less ink, are easier to read, and produce sharper photocopies. One advantage of standard grid paper is that it is slightly less expensive (see Figure 3-14).

The standard paper speed for the ECG machine is 25 mm/sec. Be sure your ECG machine is set at this speed unless ordered otherwise. If you run the machine at any speed other than 25 mm/sec, be certain to note this on the ECG results. Prior to performing an ECG, make sure the machine has enough paper to record the results. Each machine has a paper loading procedure that you should become familiar with. Many of the machines warn you when the paper is nearly gone by making a red mark across the bottom of the tracing (see Figure 3-15). Read the manufacturer's directions for

Figure 3-15 While performing an ECG, a thick red line at the bottom of the graph paper indicates that the paper needs to be changed.

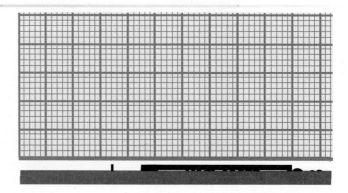

specific instructions on how to change the ECG machine paper. Keep a supply of paper on the ECG cart in case you run out of paper in the patient's room or examination room.

Measurements

The ECG graph paper consists of precisely spaced horizontal and vertical lines. The horizontal readings represent time, measured in millimeters (mm). The vertical readings measure voltage, indicated in millivolts (mV). The heavy lines form boxes that are 5 mm by 5 mm in size. The smallest box on the graph paper represents 0.04 second in time and 1 mm or 0.1 mV in voltage. At the normal paper speed, one second equals 25 mm, or five heavy lines. Therefore, each vertical heavy line represents 0.20 second. Two large boxes represent 10 mm, which equals 1 centimeter (cm). ECG machines must be calibrated so that 1 cm = 1 mV. Each heavy line horizontally represents 5 mm or .5 mV (see Figure 3-16). A calibration mark should always be verified on the left-hand side of the ECG before printing.

Calculating Heart Rate

A quick look at the ECG tracing can give you an idea of the heart rate. The more space between the QRS complexes, the slower the heart rate. The less space between the QRS complexes, the faster the heart rate. A more accurate approximation can be done with a variety of methods. For a regular rhythm,

Figure 3-16 The ECG paper will provide measurement for both time and voltage. Note that each small box is either 0.1mV in voltage or 0.04 seconds in time.

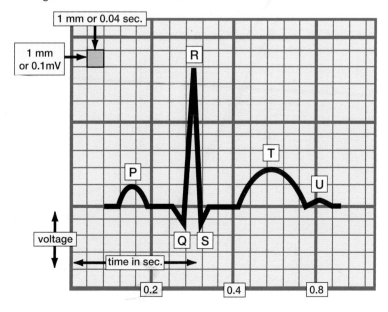

Five vertical heavy lines or boxes = 1 second

One vertical heavy line or box = 0.2 seconds

Smallest vertical line or box = 0.04 seconds

Two large horizontal heavy lines or boxes = 1 mV

TABLE 3-2 Calculating Heart Rates with Measurement of the R-R Interval

Large Boxes Between Two R Waves	Seconds Between Beats	Heart Beats per Minute
1	0.2	300
2	0.4	150
3	0.6	100
4	0.8	75
5	1.0	60
6	1.2	50

the R-R wave method is useful. For regular or irregular rhythms, you can use the 6-second or 1500 method.

For the R-R method, when you are running the ECG at 25 mm/sec, there are 300 large boxes in a 1-minute strip. (This method is sometimes called the 300 method.) If the rhythm is regular, you need to first determine the number of large boxes between two R waves on the ECG tracing. This number should be divided into 300. For example, if there were five boxes between the R waves, the heart rate would be 300 divided by 5, which equals 60 beats per minute. Table 3-2 provides the approximate heart rates based on this method of calculation. See Figure 3-17 for calculating heart rates using the R-R wave method.

A second method for approximating the heart rate is called the 6-second method. First, identify a 6-second section of the tracing. The ECG paper is usually marked at 3-second intervals on the top or bottom of the strip with a vertical line. You will need to view two sections or 30 boxes, horizontally. Second, count the number of complete complexes seen in one 6-second interval. Each complex must include the P, QRS, and T waves. The complex should not be counted unless complete. Third, multiply the number of

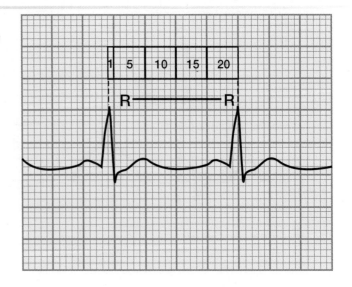

Figure 3-17 To estimate the heart rate with the R-R wave method, count the number of large boxes between two R waves and divide into 300. In this figure there are four full boxes between the R waves for an estimated rate of 75.

Figure 3-18 To estimate the heart rate with the six-second method, locate a six-second section of the ECG rhythm strip (each small black line or heavy red mark at the top of the strip indicates 15 boxes or three seconds), count the number of complete complexes in this section, then multiply the number of complexes by 10. In this figure, 8 complete complexes equal an estimated heart rate of 80.

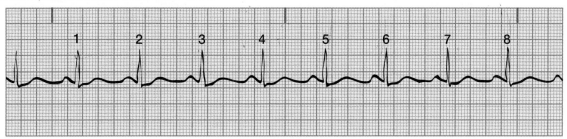

complexes by 10 to determine the estimated heart rate. This method can be used when the rhythm is irregular (see Figure 3-18 and "Troubleshooting—*Counting the Heart Rate*").

A third method of calculating the heart rate is the 1500 method. This is named such because in a 1-minute interval there are 1500 small squares. To use this method, you should count the number of small squares between two consecutive R waves and then divide that number into 1500. For example, if you count 25 small squares between two R waves, you will divide that by 1500 (1500 ÷ 25 = 60). The heart rate would be 60 beats per minute (see Figure 3-19).

Troubleshooting **Counting the Heart Rate**

When calculating the heart rate by counting the complexes in the 6-second interval, count the complete complexes only. If there is a portion of a complex at each end of the 6-second section you are using, find another section on the tracing to view. Never count incomplete complexes; this will make your results inaccurate.

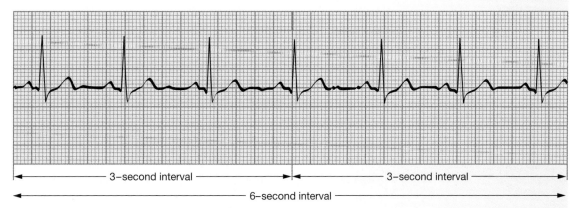

Multiply the number of QRS complexes or P waves by 10

What is the number of complexes in the above 6-second interval? What is the heart rate?

_____

_____

Figure 3-19 Using the 1500 method count the number of small boxes between two R waves and divide into 1500. In this example there are 38 small boxes. 1500 ÷ 38 = 40 beats per minute.

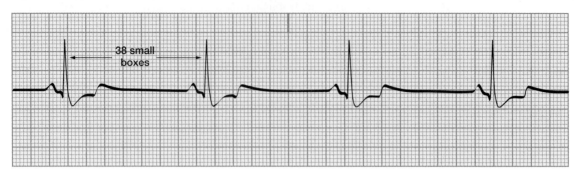

 Checkpoint Question 3-5

1. When the paper speed is 25 mm/sec, there are how many boxes per minute?

_____

_____

Answer the preceding question and complete the "ECG Graph Paper" activity on the student CD under Chapter 3 before you proceed to the next section.

Chapter Summary

- Three types of leads are used to produce the ECG; standard, augmented, and chest leads.
- Standard leads are bipolar, meaning they measure electricity in two directions. Augmented leads are unipolar because they measure toward one electrode on the body. Chest leads record activity between six points on the chest and within the heart.
- A single channel ECG records 12 leads individually, and a multichannel ECG monitors all 12 leads and usually records three at a time.
- The ECG machine has three basic functions; input, signal processing, and output display.
- The controls for the ECG machine include the speed, gain, artifact filter, LCD display, heart rate limits, standardization, and the lead selector.
- Most common ECG machines include a keyboard and lead wires for input, a small machine that processes the ECG signal, and an LCD display and paper for output.
- Various types of disposable electrodes are used depending upon the equipment and type of ECG being recorded.
- ECG graph paper has boxes that are 5 mm by 5 mm and indicate 0.04 second in time horizontally and 0.1 mV in voltage vertically.
- There are three common ways to calculate the heart rate including the R-R (300) method, the 6-second method, and the 1500 method.

Chapter Review

Matching I

Match the name of each of the following leads with their lead type. Place the correct letter on the line provided.

_____ 1. V1

_____ 2. aVR

_____ 3. lead I

_____ 4. lead II

_____ 5. aVL

_____ 6. V3

_____ 7. V4

_____ 8. V6

_____ 9. aVF

_____ 10. lead III

_____ 11. V2

_____ 12. V5

a. standard limb lead

b. augmented lead

c. precordial lead

Matching II

Match these terms related to the ECG with their definitions. Place the correct letter on the line provided.

_____ 13. single-channel

_____ 14. speed

_____ 15. input

_____ 16. gain

_____ 17. lead

_____ 18. multichannel

_____ 19. mV

_____ 20. mm

_____ 21. signal processing

_____ 22. electrode

_____ 23. output display

a. disposable sensors that receive the electrical activity of the heart

b. changes the size of the ECG tracing

c. data that is entered into an ECG machine

d. indicates time on the ECG tracing

e. conductor wire attached to the ECG machine

f. ability to record more than one lead tracing at a time

g. indicates voltage on the ECG tracing

h. displays the tracing for the electrical activity of the heart

i. amplifies the electrical impulse and converts to mechanical action

j. records one lead tracing at a time

k. controls the speed of the paper during an ECG tracing

Multiple Choice

Circle the correct answer.

24. ECG machines have three basic functions. They are
    a. input, signal processing, and output display.
    b. input, standardization, and output display.
    c. multichannel, single-channel, and signal processing.
    d. standardization, input display, and output display.

25. To perform an ECG with accuracy, the best source to obtain specific information about the machine is
    a. the policy and procedure manual.
    b. the manufacturer's directions.
    c. your supervisor.
    d. your textbook.

26. The type of electrodes most commonly used are _____ and are used _____.
    a. disposable, more than once
    b. reusable, more than once
    c. disposable, once
    d. reusable, once

27. "Bipolar leads" means that
    a. One electrode is placed on the chest and the machine arbitrarily places one behind the person.
    b. Both positive and negative electrodes are placed on the patient's body.
    c. Einthoven's triangle is not used.
    d. One of the leg limbs is used while the machine augments the rhythm.

28. What is the purpose of the LCD display?
    a. To allow entry and display of patient information
    b. To show the results of the ECG
    c. To sound alarms and errors
    d. To assist the patient to understand the procedure

29. The "multichannel ECG" indicates that
    a. You enter all the data into the machine prior to running a tracing.
    b. Three or more leads are recorded at one time.
    c. You do not have to mount each lead separately.
    d. All of the above.

30. What is the standard paper speed?
    a. 25 mm/sec
    b. 50 mm/sec
    c. 0.25 mm/sec
    d. 0.50 mm/sec

31. Which of the following is not a type of lead?
    a. Standard
    b. Augmented
    c. Input
    d. Precordial

32. Artifact filter helps obtain a clear ECG tracing by
    a. reducing artifact or abnormal marks on the ECG tracing.
    b. always ensuring accurate readings by the computer.
    c. always recognizing that the patient has a pacemaker.
    d. all of the above.

33. Computerized interpretation
    a. can be used for actual diagnostic interpretation.
    b. never has to be validated by a physician.
    c. must always be validated by a physician.
    d. none of the above.

34. The horizontal reading on the ECG paper represents _____, and the vertical readings represent _____.
    a. voltage, time
    b. time, height
    c. time, voltage
    d. voltage, millivolts

35. Which lead tracing must be augmented by the ECG machine to be able to see the different ECG waveforms?
    a. Lead I
    b. Lead II
    c. Lead V6
    d. Lead aVF

36. The Einthoven triangle is formed by using the following placement sites.
    a. Right arm, left arm, left leg
    b. Right arm, left leg, right leg
    c. Right arm, middle of chest, left leg
    d. None of the above

Matching III

Match the size of the line with the time on the tracing at 25 mm/soc paper speed. Place your answer in the space provided. Note: a heavy line or box is 5 small boxes.

_____ 37. five heavy lines or boxes   **a.** 1 second

_____ 38. one vertical heavy line or box   **b.** 0.04 second

_____ 39. smallest vertical line or box   **c.** 0.2 second

Matching IV

Match the lead wire and its color. Place your answer in the space provided.

_____ 40. left leg (LL)   **a.** green

_____ 41. right arm (RA)   **b.** white

_____ 42. right leg (RL)   **c.** black

_____ 43. left arm (LA)   **d.** red

Label the Parts

44. Label the lead tracings that produce the Einthoven triangle.

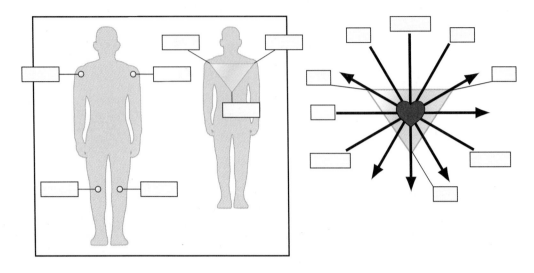

45. Label the measurements indicated on the following figure.

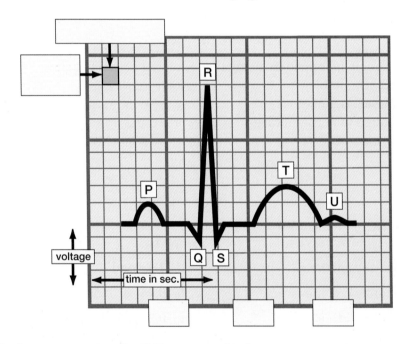

46–47. Estimate the heart rate using the R-R wave method.

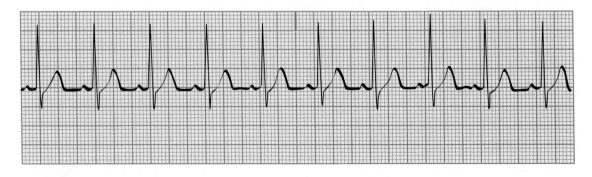

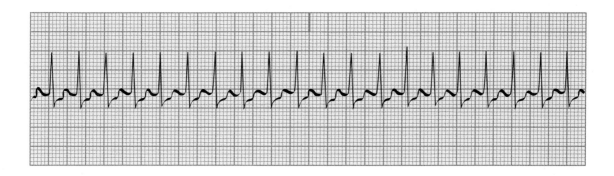

48–49. Estimate the heart rate using the 6-second method.

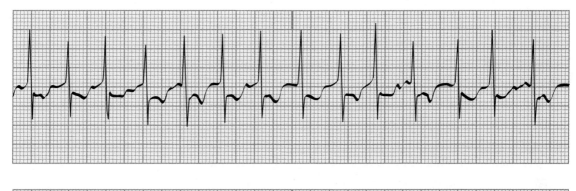

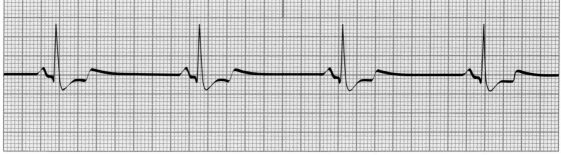

50–51. Determine the heart rate using the 1500 method.

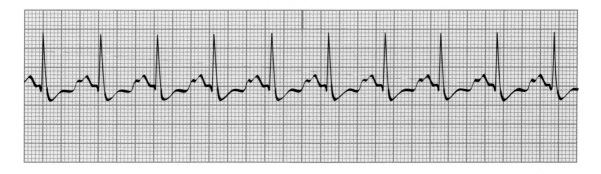

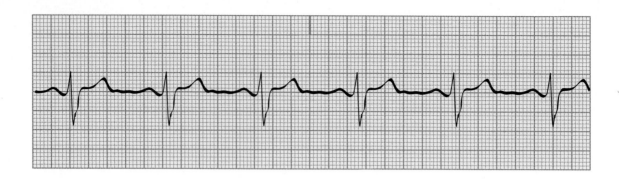

What Should You Do? *Critical Thinking Application*

Read the following situations and use your critical thinking skills to determine how you would handle each. Write your answer in detail in the space provided.

52. When you start to perform an ECG on a patient, you notice a red line along the bottom of the ECG paper. What should you do?

_____

_____

53. When preparing to do an ECG, you find an open package of disposable electrodes on top of the ECG cart. Would you use these electrodes? Why or why not?

_____

_____

54. You are preparing to attach the electrodes and lead wires for a 12-lead ECG. You are unable to read the letters on each of the lead wires. You place the electrodes and lead wires, but when you run the tracing it looks like a bunch of scratches. What do you think the problem is and how would you solve it?

_____

_____

55. When performing a 12-lead ECG, you notice that the tracing line is very thick and hard to view. In addition, one of the leads does not record properly. What would you do?

_____

_____

Get Connected *Internet Activity*

Visit the McGraw-Hill Higher Education Online Learning Center *Electrocardiography for Health Care Personnel* Web site at **www.mhhe.com/healthcareskills** to complete the following activity.
Visit the Web site NobelPrize.org to learn more about how the ECG is produced. Read the article, then click the link to play the "Electrocardiogram Game" and practice your skills as an ECG technician.

Using the Student CD

Now that your have completed the material in the chapter text, return to the student CD and complete any chapter activities you have not yet done. Practice your terminology with the "Key Term Concentration" game. Review the chapter material with the "Spin the Wheel" game. Take the final chapter test and complete the troubleshooting question and email or print your results to document your proficiency for this chapter.

Performing an ECG

4

Learning Outcomes

- Demonstrate proficiency in preparing the patient, room, and equipment for an ECG.
- Discuss what to do in the event that the patient refuses an ECG.
- Demonstrate the proper procedure for the application of the electrodes and lead wires for a 12-lead and continuous monitoring ECG.
- Identify at least three ways to prevent infection during the ECG procedure.
- Identify at least three ways to provide for safety during the ECG procedure.
- Identify two measures to ensure HIPAA compliance while performing ECGs.
- Identify types of artifact and how to prevent or correct them.
- Demonstrate the proper procedure for recording and reporting a 12-lead ECG.
- Describe the procedure for mounting a single-lead ECG tracing correctly.
- Compare and contrast the adult and pediatric ECG procedures.
- Troubleshoot special patient circumstances when performing an ECG.
- Clean and care for the ECG equipment.

Key Terms

AC (alternating current) interference

angle of Louis

anterior axillary line

artifact

complexes

dextrocardia

intercostal space (ICS)

midaxillary line

midclavicular line

midscapular line

paraspinal line

posterior axillary line

seizure

somatic tremor

stat

suprasternal notch

wandering baseline

4.1 Introduction

Now that you understand how the ECG is used, the anatomy of the heart, and the electrocardiograph, the next step is to record an ECG. The ECG experience should be pleasant to the patient and not produce anxiety. The ECG procedure must be done correctly and the tracing must be accurate. This chapter will provide you with information necessary to record an ECG professionally, without error, while keeping the patient as comfortable as possible.

✓ Checkpoint Question 4-1

1. Name four important aspects of performing an ECG.

_____

_____

4.2 Preparation for the ECG Procedure

Prior to performing the ECG, you will need to prepare the room. Certain conditions in the room where the ECG is to be performed should be considered. For example, electrical currents in the room can interfere with the tracing. If possible, choose a room away from other electrical equipment and x-ray machines. If electrical equipment is in the room, turn off any that you can during the tracing. The ECG machine should be placed away from other sources of electrical currents such as wires or cords.

An ECG must be ordered by a physician and an order form must be completed prior to the procedure. This form may be called a requisition or consult and should be placed in the patient's record. It should include why the ECG was ordered and the following identifying information:

- Patient name, identification number or medical record number, and birth date
- Location, date, and time of recording
- Patient age, sex, race, and cardiac medications the patient is currently taking
- Weight and height
- Any special condition or position of the patient during the recording

If this information is not included on the requisition or consult, you should ask the patient or find the information in the patient's record.

Cardiac Medications

Certain cardiac medications can change the ECG tracing. Determine if your patient is on any cardiac medications prior to the ECG procedure; and, if so, inform the physician and write the names of the medications on the ECG report. See Appendix B for some common cardiac medications.

Many facilities have computerized systems. The ECG order is frequently entered through this system. Entering the patient identifying information into the computer will produce the order form and generate patient charges. If your facility does not have a computer system, the information should be handwritten on the order form, consult, or requisition, whichever your facility uses.

The patient identifying information should also be entered through the LCD panel on the ECG machine prior to the recording. If the ECG machine does not allow you to enter the information or there isn't time due to an emergency situation, you should write it on the completed ECG. Most importantly, all information should be written or entered accurately no matter what type of ECG machine or order system you are using.

Before beginning the procedure, make sure the ECG machine has a good supply of paper loaded in it. If a red line is seen across the bottom of the last tracing, you should replace the paper in the ECG machine before beginning. This should be done prior to taking the ECG machine to the room where the patient is located. Review the operator's manual or consult with your supervisor if you are unsure how to insert the new ream of paper. Since ECG machines and paper differ, the operator's manual is a valuable source of information. Typically, the single-channel ECG machines use a thin roll and multichannel ECG machines use wider, fan-folded type paper. Each ECG machine will have a release button or lever that will open the ECG equipment for the paper to be inserted. Place the paper inside the machine correctly. Thread it through the rollor to the outside of the machine and align. Close the paper-loading compartment and run the machine to check for proper functioning and alignment (see Figure 4-1).

Checkpoint Question 4-2

1. What information must be included on the ECG requisition?

_____

_____

Answer the preceding question and complete the "Preparation for the ECG Procedure" activity on the student CD under Chapter 4 before you proceed to the next section.

Figure 4-1 Make sure the ECG paper is properly loaded and aligned before recording an ECG.

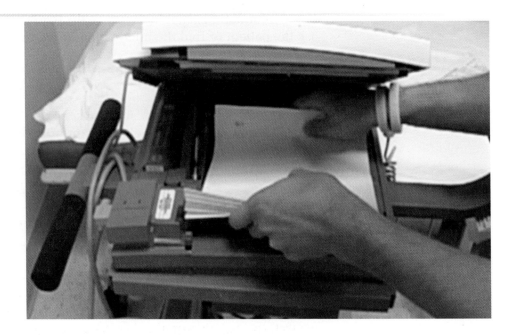

4.3 Communicating with the Patient

Prior to performing any procedure, always ensure that you are performing the procedure on the correct patient. Correctly identifying the patient is the first step in ensuring that you are providing patient safety. You should always identify the name, verify the name with some form of identification, and ensure that it is the right patient for the procedure. The Joint Commission on Accreditation of Healthcare Organizations (JCAHO) has stated that every patient must be identified by two forms of identification. This can be a photo ID, the patient stating his or her name, a medical record number, and/or verification of the patient's birth date with the patient statement. If the patient's information is incorrect, verify with your immediate supervisor for the next steps.

Introduce yourself by stating your name and job title. Ask the patient to state his or her name. Check the name on the patient identification band or patient's chart to verify the information. To ensure it is the correct patient, ask the patient to state his or her birth date. Often patients have similar names but their birth dates and medical record number will distinguish the correct patient.

After you verify that you have the correct patient, explain what you are about to do. State "I am going to perform an electrocardiogram on you today. Have you ever had an ECG done before?" Stating both ECG and electrocardiogram helps the patient relate that they are the same. If the patient has not had an ECG, explain the procedure in more detail. Assure the patient that the procedure is harmless and painless. Avoid using words that may frighten the patient such as *electricity* or *wires*. Patients, particularly children, who have not had an ECG before may be afraid of the machine and wires. The patient should be relaxed and comfortable. Maintaining a calm, competent manner and answering the patient's questions will help the patient relax.

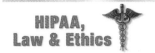
Legal Record

The ECG is part of the medical record. Enter the patient information thoroughly and accurately. Remember, the patient's medical record can be used as part of a medical professional liability case.

If the patient refuses an ECG, determine the cause of the refusal. Some people may have fear or concern about the procedure. Provide any information or reassurance the patient may need. Frequently, patients see the wires and think the machine will shock them. Be sure you explain carefully that you are only going to measure the electricity that is already inside their body. If the patient still refuses, notify your supervisor; the patient's reason for refusal must be documented.

In preparing for an ECG, provide the patient with privacy by pulling a curtain around the bed or closing the examination room door. Because many patients are fearful and/or feel they lack privacy, inform them that closing the door or curtain is for their privacy. The patient should remove any clothing above the waist. Provide the patient with a drape, such as a sheet or blanket. The patient may also wear a hospital-type gown with the opening in the front. The patient should remove any jewelry or items that would interfere with the electrode placement or touch the electrodes. This may include necklaces, watches, bracelets, belt buckles, or ankle bracelets. In addition, all electronic devices need to be turned off and removed from the patient. These include things such as cell phones, PDAs, MP3 players, or beepers.

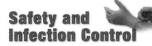

**Patient Education &
Communication**

Explain the Procedure

Remember, even if a patient is not able to respond, he or she may still hear you. Always explain the procedure before beginning the ECG.

**Safety and
Infection Control**

Proper Patient Identification

You must always check the patient's name and medical record or patient identification number and verify it with the patient's birth date prior to performing any procedure on a patient.

The patient should be positioned as comfortably as possible on his or her back and should remain relaxed and still throughout the procedure. To ensure comfort, place a small pillow under the patient's head and an extra pillow under the knees, if preferred.

The position of the patient is important during an ECG. Expose the patient's chest and extremities where you will be placing the leads. If possible, work from the left side of the bed or exam table, since most of the electrodes and leads are placed on the left side of the chest. Ensure that the arms and legs are supported on the exam table or bed. Take care to provide for privacy by using the blanket or sheet to drape the patient. It is especially important to drape a female patient's breasts for comfort and to prevent embarrassment. A sheet or blanket will also keep the patient warm and prevent chills. Chills may produce shivers that could interfere with the tracing. Make sure that the bed or exam table is not touching the wall or any electrical equipment and that the patient is not touching any metal. If the exam table is especially narrow or the patient is large, you may use blankets, sheets, or pillows to prevent direct contact with the rails, thus reducing the potential for artifact.

Checkpoint Question 4-3

1. What should you indicate to the patient when closing the door or pulling the curtain before performing an ECG?

_____

_____

Answer the preceding question and complete the "Communicating with the Patient" activity on the student CD under Chapter 4 before you proceed to the next section.

4.4 Identifying Anatomical Landmarks

Once you have properly positioned the patient on the bed or exam table, you will need to place the electrodes on the chest and limbs. In order to place the chest electrodes for the ECG, you must have an understanding of the anatomy and certain landmarks on the chest. Each chest lead, V1 to V6, must be placed on the correct site on the chest. These sites can be identified by knowing the underlying bones and a set of imaginary lines on the exterior of the chest.

The bones of the chest include the clavicle, the sternum, and the ribs. The imaginary lines include the midclavicular line, the midaxillary line, and the anterior axillary line. On most patients, the **midclavicular line** starts in the center of the clavicle and passes vertically through the nipple line. The **anterior axillary line** starts in the front of the axilla and runs down the left side of the chest. The **midaxillary line** starts in the middle of the axilla (armpit) and runs down the side of the chest.

Other sites on the chest you must be able to locate include the intercostal spaces, suprasternal notch, and the angle of Louis. To feel the **intercostal space (ICS)**, or space between two ribs, locate the sternum. Press your fingers to the edge of the sternum on the left or right side. The outer edge of the sternum is known as the sternal border. Between each connected rib you should feel a dip or dent. Feeling as close to the sternal border as possible will make it easier. The **suprasternal notch** is the dip you feel at the base of the neck just above where the clavicle attaches to the sternum. The **angle of Louis** is a ridge about an inch or so below the suprasternal notch. It is where the main part of the sternum and the manubrium (top of the sternum) attach to the right and left of the "angle of Louis" are the second ribs. Below each rib is the corresponding intercostal space (ICS) (see Figure 4-2).

Figure 4-2 Anatomical landmarks for chest lead placement.

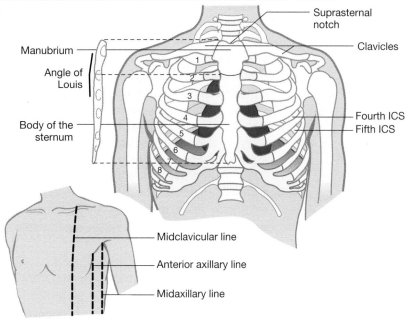

- Suprasternal notch
- Clavicles
- Manubrium
- Angle of Louis
- Body of the sternum
- Fourth ICS
- Fifth ICS
- Midclavicular line
- Anterior axillary line
- Midaxillary line

Checkpoint Questions 4-4

1. Which anatomical landmark starts in the middle of the axilla and runs down the side of the chest?

_____

_____

2. Where is the angle of Louis?

_____

Answer the preceding questions and complete the "Identifying Anatomical Landmarks" activity on the student CD under Chapter 4 before you proceed to the next section.

4.5 Applying the Electrodes and Leads

Before applying the electrodes on the chest, make sure the skin at the sites is clean and dry. Remove any lotion or oil from the skin with alcohol wipes or soap and water. You may use electrolyte pads to prep the skin. If the patient has a great deal of chest hair, you may also need to shave small areas of the chest so the electrodes will adhere to the skin properly. Small areas of the chest may be shaved, but it is preferred to clip the hair instead of shaving. This prevents the patient from scratching the electrode site as the hair grows in (see Table 4-1).

Start by applying the V1 electrode. First locate the angle of Louis; then locate the second rib, which is adjacent to this landmark. Each intercostal space is felt between the ribs with the corresponding intercostal space below the rib location. The fourth intercostal space is the dent you feel between the fourth and fifth ribs. Chest lead V1 is placed at the right sternal border

TABLE 4-1 Applying Leads Correctly

- Choose a flat, nonmuscular area.
- Use the forearms and ankles for the limb leads.
- Alternate sites include the upper arms near the shoulders (deltoids) and upper legs.
- Prep the skin with an electrolyte pad, if available.
- When necessary, cleanse the electrode sites with an alcohol pad, mild soap and water, or electrolyte pad.
- Dry the skin completely before applying the electrodes.
- If the patient is diaphoretic (sweaty) consider using antiperspirant, tincture of benzoin, or mastisol to help pads remain adhered to the patient's skin.
- Shave the hair from the site only if necessary such as during an emergency.
- Clip hair, instead of shaving. Use tape to remove cut hairs.

at this location. V2 should be placed at the fourth intercostal space on the left sternal border. Skip V3 and place V4 next. V4 is placed at the fifth intercostal space on the left midclavicular line. Locate the site of the intersection between the fifth intercostal space and the midclavicular line. In young people, this site is directly below the nipple. Now place V3 midway between V2 and V4. Continuing in the fifth intercostal space, place V5 at the anterior axillary line. Place V6 in the fifth intercostal space, at the midaxillary line (see Figure 4-3 and Table 4-2).

The procedure is the same when placing the chest electrodes on a female. If the patient has large breasts, you can ask the patient to move her

Figure 4-3 Chest lead placement.

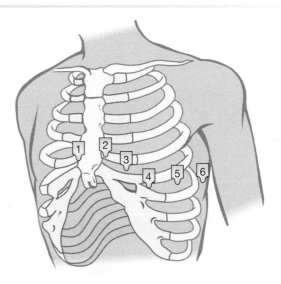

TABLE 4-2 Chest Lead Placement

V1 Fourth intercostal space, right sternal border
V2 Fourth intercostal space, left sternal border
V3 Halfway between V2 and V4
V4 Fifth intercostal space at the midclavicular line
V5 Fifth intercostal space, at the anterior axillary line
V6 Fifth intercostal space, at the midaxillary line

own breasts (if able); or, using the back of your hand, simply lift the left breast and place the electrodes in the closest position possible. Leads V3, V4, and V5 will be the most affected by breast tissue. Electrodes should be placed as close as possible to the proper placement without placing the electrodes directly on the breast tissue, because breast tissue is a poor conductor of electricity.

The limb electrodes are placed on the forearm or upper arms and the inside of the lower legs. You should pick a fleshy area with the least amount of hair. If the placement of the arm leads on the patient's forearm is not possible due to injury, amputation, IV placement, casts, or otherwise, you should chose a different site. The alternate site of placement for arm leads is on the deltoids (shoulders). The leads should be placed on the same site on each arm and should match. For example, if a patient has a cast or an IV on the left forearm, you will need to move *both* left and right electrodes to the shoulders.

Troubleshooting **The Midclavicular Line**

When locating the midclavicular line for chest lead placement, keep in mind that the midclavicular line does not always run directly through the nipple line. This is most often the case with obese patients or females with large breasts.

When applying the V4 electrode to a patient who weighs 326 pounds, you have difficulty finding the midclavicular line. What should you do?

_____

_____

When placement of the leg leads on the patient's lower legs or ankles is not possible, the alternate site for placement is on the upper legs. They should be placed as close to the trunk as possible. This may be necessary when the patient is an amputee or has an injury or bandage on one of the lower legs. The leads should be placed at the same site on each leg: if you place one lead above the knee on the left, then the right leg lead should also be placed above the knee.

After all of the electrodes have been properly positioned, you must attach the lead cable wires. Identify the correct cable for each electrode based on color and letter abbreviations. For example, the chest leads are marked V1 to V6 (see Figure 4-4). The correct cable must be attached to the corresponding electrode to ensure an accurate tracing. With some ECG machines, the electrode wires are placed with the wire connection toward the same direction typically away from the direction of the feet. When using electrodes with tabs on which the alligator-type clips are used, chest and arm electrodes are placed with the tabs pointing downward toward the feet and the lower extremity electrodes pointing toward the head. Utilizing this technique reduces tension on the electrodes and provides a more "clean" or artifact-free tracing. Ultimately, refer to the manufacturer's directions in the operator's manual for the most optimum placement technique recommended for your equipment. In all cases, the electrodes should be secure and the lead wires should be supported.

Figure 4-4 Color and letter coding identify the lead wires for an ECG machine.

Identifying Lead Wires

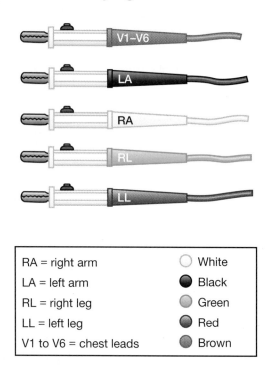

RA = right arm	⚪ White
LA = left arm	⚫ Black
RL = right leg	🟢 Green
LL = left leg	🔴 Red
V1 to V6 = chest leads	🟤 Brown

The ECG lead wire cables should follow the contours of the body when attached to the ECG electrodes. Avoid looping the wires outside of the body and check each wire once it is connected to ensure that there is no tension on the electrodes or leads. Individual loops may be used to take up slack and prevent looping outside the body, thus reducing tension on the electrode (see Figure 4-5).

Figure 4-5 Correct (left) and incorrect (right) lead cable placement. Avoid looping the wires outside the body and check each wire once it is connected to ensure that there is no tension on the electrodes or leads.

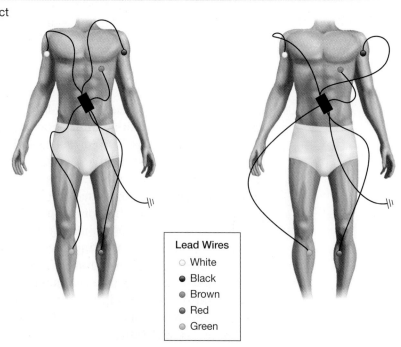

Lead Wires
- ⚪ White
- ⚫ Black
- 🟤 Brown
- 🔴 Red
- 🟢 Green

1. How can you be certain you are attaching the lead wires to the electrodes properly?

_____

_____

 Answer the preceding question and complete the "Applying the Electrodes and Leads" activity on the student CD under Chapter 4 before you proceed to the next section.

4.6 Safety and Infection Control

When performing an ECG, you must always follow precautions. You must practice universal or standard precautions at all times. These precautions are followed in all situations in which job exposure to blood or body fluids is likely. Wash your hands carefully before and after the procedure to prevent transfer of microorganisms. Wear gloves if there is a risk of exposure to the patient's blood or other body fluids.

In the hospital, you will need to follow additional precautions for patients in isolation. Depending on the type of isolation, masks, eye protection, and gowns may also be necessary when entering the room. Follow the facility's policy and the guidelines provided in Table 4-3. You should know standard precautions related to all hospitalized patients and maintain them throughout the procedure. As a rule, it is better to wear gloves even if it is not necessary. Do not forget to wash your hands or perform hand hygiene before putting on the gloves and after removing them.

Patient Education & Communication

Relocating Electrodes

When moving the electrodes to a different location due to an amputation or bandages, you should document this on the 12-lead ECG recording.

General safety guidelines and safety measures specific to the ECG procedure must also be practiced. Before beginning the procedure, you must identify, verify, and ensure that you are performing the procedure on the correct patient. Use two forms of identification, for example, the patient's name, birth date, and/or medical record number. Then you should raise the side rail on the unattended side of the patient's bed or exam table. If the patient is on an exam table, have him or her lie down and pull the extension out for his or her legs and feet. Prior to performing the ECG, check to be sure that the grounding prong is securely attached to the plug. Plug the machine in securely. Ensure that the bed or exam table is not touching the wall or any electrical equipment. Be sure that the patient is not touching the bed or exam table frame or safety rail. Always check the insulation on the lead wires for cracks before each use. Ensure that all electronic devices the patient may have are turned off and removed from the patient (see Table 4-4 and Table 4-5).

TABLE 4-3 Infection Control Guidelines for Isolation of Hospitalized Patients

In addition to standard precautions, follow these guidelines and the policy of your place of employment to prevent the spread of infections.

Airborne Precautions

For patients known or suspected to be infected with microorganisms transmitted by minute airborne droplets:

- Use a private room that has monitored negative air.
- Keep the room door closed and the patient in the room.
- Wear respiratory protection when entering the room of a patient with known or suspected infectious pulmonary tuberculosis.
- Wear special HEPA N-95, N-99, or N-100 masks when entering the room.
- Do not enter the room of a patient known or suspected to have rubeola or varicella if you are susceptible; if you must enter the room, wear respiratory protection.
- Limit the movement and transport of patients from the room to essential purposes only.
- Place a surgical mask on the patient, if transport or movement is necessary.

Droplet Precautions

For patients known or suspected to be infected with microorganisms transmitted by droplets that can be generated by the patient during coughing, sneezing, talking, or the performance of procedures:

- Place patient in a private room (special air handling and ventilation are not necessary and the door may remain open).
- Wear a mask when working within 3 feet of the patient.
- Limit the movement and transport of the patient from the room to essential purposes only.
- Use a mask on the patient, if transport or movement is necessary.

Contact Precautions

For patients known or suspected to be infected or colonized with microorganisms that can be transmitted by direct or indirect contact (direct contact includes hand or skin-to-skin contact that occurs when performing patient care that requires touching the patient's dry skin; indirect contact includes touching environmental surfaces or patient-care items in the patient's environment):

- Place patients in a private room.
- Wear gloves according to standard precautions.
- Wear gloves when entering the room and while providing patient care.
- Change gloves after having contact with infective material that may contain high concentrations of microorganisms such as feces and wound drainage.
- Remove gloves before leaving the patient's room.
- Wash hands immediately.
- Do not touch potentially contaminated environmental surfaces or items in the patient's room after glove removal.
- All equipment must be disinfected after entering the patient's room. The 12-lead ECG machine needs to be wiped down immediately

TABLE 4-4 Maintaining Safety During an ECG

- Check that the grounding prong is securely attached the plug.
- Plug the machine in securely making sure the cord is not separating from the receptacle.
- Ensure that the power cord insulation is intact.
- Remove the plug by pulling it out by the prong connection, not by pulling on the electrical cord.
- Raise the bed to a working height and return to low position when completed.
- Keep the side rail up on the opposite side of the bed or exam table.
- Perform hand hygiene and wear gloves or other personal protective equipment as required.

TABLE 4-5 Troubleshooting Techniques During an ECG

- Perform and ensure good skin preparation.
- Use fresh electrodes and clean clips.
- Make sure personal electrical devices are turned off and removed from the patient.
- Ensure that the bed or examination table is not touching the wall or any electrical equipment.
- Ensure that the patient is not touching the frame, side rail, or any metal part of the bed or examination table.
- Always check the insulation on the lead wires for cracks before use.
- Ensure that there is not stress on the lead wires or electrodes.

Prepare the patient for the procedure by first ensuring privacy and providing for the patient's safety and comfort during the ECG. The patient's door or curtain should be closed and the patient's clothing appropriately removed and draped for privacy. Assist him or her to a comfortable position in which to dress. After the procedure, you should clean the lead wires, leads, and machine. If you performed an ECG on a patient in isolation or with a contagious disease, you will need to clean the equipment properly to prevent the spread of infection. Observe the guidelines at your place of employment and the manufacturer's directions for the correct cleaning technique. Once you have completed the entire procedure, including cleanup, you should wash your hands. Remember to thank the patient and ask if he or she needs any further assistance.

Checkpoint Questions 4-6

1. Name at least three things to do to ensure safety during an ECG.

   _____

   _____

2. Name at least three troubleshooting techniques during an ECG.

   _____

   _____

 Answer the preceding questions and complete the "Safety and Infection Control" activity on the student CD under Chapter 4 before you proceed to the next section.

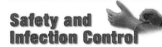 **Safety and Infection Control**

Isolation Precautions

There are three types of isolation identified by the Centers for Disease Control. They are airborne, droplet, and contact. Standard precautions include specific guidelines for caring for patients in isolation.

4.7 Operating the ECG Machine

Before operating the ECG machine, make sure you have done the following:

- Identify and communicate with the patient.
- Prepare the patient and the room.

- Provide for patient privacy.
- Provide for safety and infection control.
- Locate and check the equipment for functioning.
- Load the ECG graph paper, if necessary.
- Attach the electrodes and leads.

Now you should be ready to operate the ECG machine. For an automatic ECG, simply press the Run or Auto button. Check the LCD display for errors. If the ECG machine provides interpretation, it will print out along with the tracing. This process takes only about 15 to 20 seconds.

For a manual ECG machine, make sure the equipment is standardized and set to lead I. You may need to run a few **complexes** (complete ECG waveforms) and then insert a standardization mark. The mark should be set between the T wave of one complex and the P wave of the next. Follow specific directions provided in the operator's manual or according to your institutions policy and procedure.

Most ECG machines are automatic and mark the lead codes. If the equipment you are using does not, mark each code manually during the tracing. While the ECG is running, change the lead code dial, then mark each lead. You should run about 8 to 10 inches of complexes for leads I, II, and III. For the rest of the leads, 5 inches should be sufficient. Identify the recording with the patient's name, the date, and other required information. This is usually entered into the LCD display prior to the recording. You may need to mount the tracing upon completion of the ECG. Mounting the ECG is discussed later in this chapter under "Reporting ECG Results."

Checkpoint Question 4-7

1. If you are running a manual ECG tracing, how long of a tracing do you need to run for leads, I, II, and III?

_____

_____

 Answer the preceding question and complete the "Operating the ECG Machine" activity on the student CD under Chapter 4 before you proceed to the next section.

4.8 Checking the ECG Tracing

Certain problems can occur when obtaining an ECG tracing. The most frequent problem is unwanted marks on the ECG. These marks are called **artifact.** The marks are not caused by the heart activity; they are caused by some other source of movement or electrical activity. When an ECG tracing has these unwanted marks, it is difficult or impossible to read. You are responsible for producing a correct tracing without artifact. In order to do this, you must first recognize artifact and then be able to eliminate it. The three most common causes of artifact are somatic tremor, wandering baseline, and AC interference (see Table 4-6 for ways to correct these causes of artifact).

TABLE 4-6 Correcting Artifact

Type of Artifact	Cause	Correction
Somatic tremor	Involuntary muscle movement: shivering, muscle tension, pain, fear	Reassure the patient, warm the patient, and encourage him or her to take slow, deep breaths.
	Voluntary movement: talking, chewing gum	Remind the patient not to make any movement during the procedure.
	Movement due to neuromuscular disorder such as Parkinson's disease	Have the patient put his or her hands, palms down, under the buttocks.
Wandering baseline	Improperly applied electrodes or poor skin preparation	Apply electrodes securely, make sure that the entire surface is in contact with the patient's skin.
	Pulling on electrodes from unsupported lead wires	Remove tension from lead wires.
	Old, corroded, or dirty electrodes or clips	Keep reusable electrodes clean; store unused disposable ones in plastic bags.
	Oil, lotion, dirt, or hair on the skin under the electrodes	Clean the skin with alcohol and gauze or an alcohol prep pad.
	Too little or dried out electrode gel	Use new disposable electrodes and store unused ones in a plastic bag; if using gel, apply plenty of new solution to electrodes.
Alternating current (AC) interference	Improper grounding	Ensure that the plug has three prongs and is plugged into a grounded electrical outlet.
	Other electrical equipment	Unplug equipment and wait until any other procedure is done, if possible.
	Lead wires crossed and not pointed toward the hands and feet	Reposition the lead wires and ensure that they follow limbs and are pointed in the proper direction.
	Electrical wiring in the walls or ceiling	Move the patient's bed away from the wall (use a 45-degree angle if necessary).
	Corroded or dirty leads	Clean the leads after each use.

Somatic Tremor

Sometimes a patient's muscles will move, either voluntarily or involuntarily, which can produce **somatic tremor,** also known as body tremor. Movement of the muscles of the body is controlled by electrical voltages. These voltages are erratic, unlike the cardiac voltage, which is consistent. Somatic tremor appears as large erratic spikes on the ECG tracing (see Figure 4-6).

Figure 4-6 Somatic tremor appears as large erratic spikes on the ECG tracing.

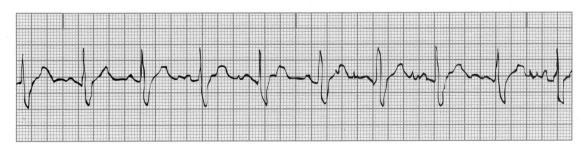

If your hospitalized patient requires daily ECGs for comparison by the physician, the ECG tracing may look different if the electrodes are placed in different sites on the chest and limbs. Each time you record an ECG on the patient, place the leads on the same site or as close as possible to the placement from the previous ECG. Some facilities will permit placing small marks on the patient to ensure that electrode placement will be consistent for multiple (serial) ECGs.

You are doing your third ECG on a patient in three days. Where should the electrodes be placed?

_____

_____

Voluntary muscle movements are due to tension, fear, gum chewing, talking, uncomfortable position, or pain. They may also be due to shivering or tense muscles. You should identify the correct cause before proceeding with the ECG. Knowing the cause will help you eliminate the artifact. Warm or reassure the patient if he or she is cold or frightened. Encourage slow, deep breaths to help calm the patient. Remind the patient to refrain from moving or talking.

Sometimes involuntary muscle movements are due to Parkinson's disease or other neuromuscular disorders. These are more difficult to control. Have patients who suffer from neuromuscular disorders put their hands, palms down, under their buttocks. This will decrease the tremor and improve the tracing. If a patient has this type of tremor, it should be recorded on the ECG tracing.

Wandering Baseline (Baseline Shift)

Wandering baseline, or baseline shift, occurs when the tracing drifts away from the center of the graph paper (see Figure 4-7). Baseline shift can have many causes. Typically, it is due to improper electrode application such as the following:

- Too loose or incorrect electrode application
- Tension or pulling on electrode lead wires
- Too little electrode gel or solution
- Old or dried out electrode gel or solution
- Corroded or dirty electrodes

Figure 4-7 Wandering baseline occurs when the baseline of the ECG tracing drifts away from the center of the ECG graph paper.

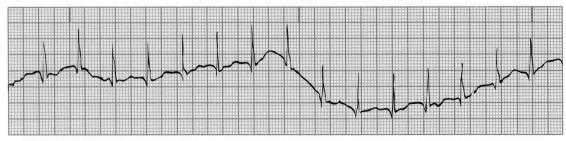

- Oil, lotion, dirt, or hair under the electrodes
- Poor or no skin preparation

To avoid problems with wandering baseline, apply the electrodes securely and make sure they are not too loose or tight. Be certain that the entire surface is in contact with the patient's skin. Check the lead wires and remove any tension from them. Use fresh electrode gel or new disposable electrodes. Make sure that previously opened electrodes have been stored in a plastic bag or container. Clean the reusable leads after each use. Clean the patient's skin carefully before applying electrodes.

Alternating Current (AC) Interference

Alternating current is normally present in all electrical equipment and wiring in the walls. Sometimes the wires can radiate or leak a small amount of energy into the immediate surrounding area. When a patient is present in this area, the patient's body may pick up some of the current. This current is then registered on the ECG and is called **AC (alternating current) interference**. AC interference will appear as uniform small spikes on the ECG tracing (see Figure 4-8).

Figure 4-8 AC (alternating current) interference appears as uniform small spikes on the ECG tracing.

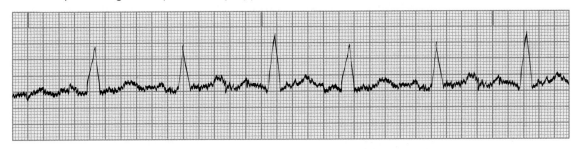

Many different things can cause AC interference artifact. These include improper grounding, other electrical equipment, lead wires crossed, and corroded or dirty electrodes. Eliminating the cause and using proper technique can prevent AC interference artifact. Eliminating sources of electrical current, ensuring proper grounding of the machine, and attaching the lead wires correctly can reduce AC interference.

The cause of AC interference is sometimes difficult to determine. You may still have AC interference even after you have checked that the machine is properly grounded, the lead wires are correct, and other equipment is turned off. In order to find the source, time permitting, you can try this technique. Run lead I, lead II, and lead III and look for interference. Evaluate each strip for interference to determine the direction or source of interference (see Table 4-7). For example, if you have the most interference in leads II and III, the source is probably near or on the left arm. You may need

TABLE 4-7 Troubleshooting AC Interference

Leads with Most AC Interference Noted	Source of Interference or Direction
Leads I and II	Right arm
Leads I and III	Left arm
Leads II and III	Left leg

to rotate the bed or exam table at a 45-degree angle away from the source. Also, do not forget the proper placement of the lead cables. They should follow the body contours and be lying flat against the skin. In addition, do not run the power cord under or over the bed or exam table. This is another possible source of electrical interference.

Artifact can also be caused by other sources. High-tension wires and transformers on a power pole and diathermy machines used to give high-frequency currents as heat treatments can cause AC interference. Electrocautery, IV pumps, feeding tubes, and x-ray machines can also interfere if they are in the room or an adjacent room. Even the electrical wires in the walls, ceiling, and floor, although they are not visible, can cause artifact. Most ECG machines have a battery that allows you to unplug and still perform the ECG. Unplugging the machine eliminates any AC interference that may be produced from the electrical outlet.

Troubleshooting

Handling a Flatline Tracing

If a flat line without deflections occurs during the tracing, it could be asystole (indicates no heart beat). Remain calm and check the patient first, since the patient is your number one concern. If the patient is able to respond, check the electrodes, lead wires, and cables.

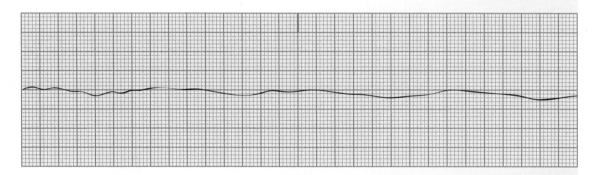

The patient's ECG tracing looks like the one pictured here. What should you do?

_____

_____

There are some additional problems you may encounter when obtaining an ECG. One example is an interrupted baseline on one or more leads. This appears as a flat line on the tracing. This could occur when a wire is not plugged in correctly or is loose. If a flat line occurs on more than one lead, it may be that the wires have been switched. Check your machine cables and connections. Ensure that the machine is set to obtain a tracing. Do not forget to check for loose or broken lead wires, which may also cause a break in the complexes or an interrupted baseline.

After troubleshooting any problem, if you cannot correct it, report it to your supervisor. If it is an AC interference problem, the biomedical engineering department, if available, may need to track down the source of the interference. It could also be that the machine requires service. In this case, the manufacturer should be called for information and assistance.

Checkpoint Questions 4-8

1. What is the cause of the following artifact?

_____

_____

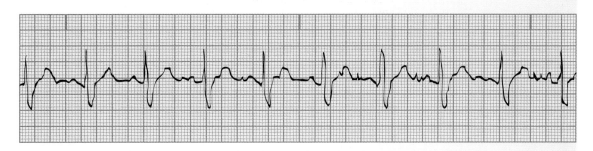

2. Name three causes of wandering baseline.

_____

_____

 Answer the preceding questions and complete the "Checking the ECG Tracing" activity on the student CD under Chapter 4 before you proceed to the next section.

4.9 Reporting ECG Results

When you have completed an ECG, use the method your facility requires for reporting the results. Check your facility policy to be certain you are placing the completed ECG tracings in the appropriate place. In many situations, you will be required to make two copies, one to be placed on the patient's chart and the other to be read by the consulting physician. In the hospital, the second copy is often taken back to the ECG department or stored on the computer for evaluation in the ECG laboratory. The second copy may also be placed in a box at the nursing station where the patient is located. In an ambulatory care facility, it may be attached to the front of the chart and/or placed on the physician's desk.

Some facilities have a computer that can read the ECG electronically and/or store it electronically in a central database for future reference. In addition, sometimes ECG tracings are faxed to other locations. These procedures require special equipment. You may be asked to perform either of these procedures. If so, you must be trained using your facility's equipment. If the ECG was ordered **stat** (immediately), you will need to give the results directly and immediately to your superior or the physician. If your supervisor is not available, place the results on top of the chart, find your supervisor, and inform him or her that the ECG has been completed. Remember, in a stat situation, the patient may have a condition that needs immediate treatment and no time should be wasted.

As previously discussed, billing is another issue to consider when reporting completion of an ECG. When you enter the data into the machine or on the designated form, it must be complete and accurate. If the patient is not charged for the procedure, this can have an adverse effect on the hospital's finances and subsequently your job. Check the facility policy to be certain you have completed the necessary steps to ensure that the patient will be charged.

In many facilities, the information is entered into a computer to be sent to the billing department. You may need to enter the patient's diagnosis, which is provided by the physician and is found on the chart. Each diagnosis has a special diagnostic code, known as an ICD-9 code. In some cases, you will need to identify the correct code when entering the information for the billing department. Using these codes helps ensure that the facility is reimbursed for the procedure.

Mounting the ECG Tracing

Single-channel ECG machines produce tracings on a single narrow strip displaying each of the 12 leads. When the tracing is recorded, each of the 12 leads should be marked so you will be able to identify them. If you are using a single-channel machine, you will need to mount the tracing so it can be evaluated. Most companies have standard mounts that require you to identify each lead and place it in the appropriate position on the mount. The single tracing can be cut into smaller segments to place on the preprinted mount. In addition, you will need to record on the mount identifying information and any special patient circumstances of the ECG procedure. Following proper mounting procedure is vital to ensure that the physician can easily review and interpret the results (see Figure 4-9).

**Checkpoint
Questions
4-9**

1. How should you report a stat ECG?

   _____

   _____

2. How should you mount a single-channel ECG?

   _____

   _____

 Answer the preceding questions and complete the "Reporting ECG Results" activity on the student CD under Chapter 4 before you proceed to the next section.

Figure 4-9 Single-channel ECG tracings must be cut into smaller segments and placed onto a cardboard mount for viewing and evaluation by the physician.

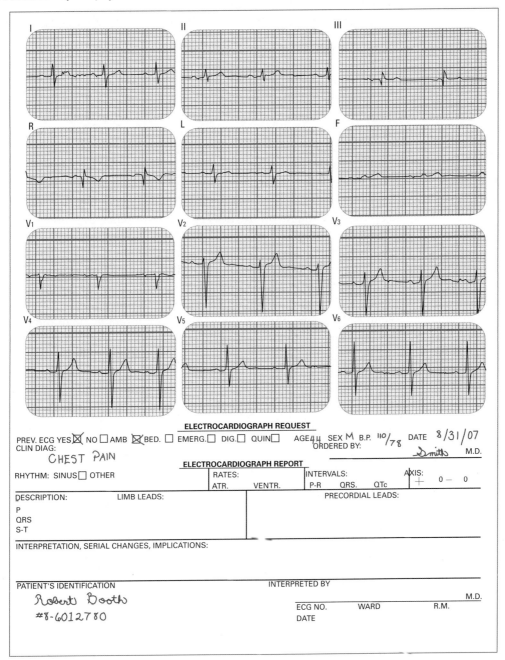

ELECTROCARDIOGRAPH REQUEST

PREV. ECG YES ☒ NO ☐ AMB ☒ BED. ☐ EMERG. ☐ DIG. ☐ QUIN ☐   AGE 44 SEX M B.P. 110/78 DATE 8/31/07

CLIN DIAG: ORDERED BY:
CHEST PAIN   Smith   M.D.

ELECTROCARDIOGRAPH REPORT

	RATES:		INTERVALS:			AXIS:	
RHYTHM: SINUS ☐ OTHER	ATR.	VENTR.	P-R	QRS	QTc	+ 0 — 0	

DESCRIPTION: LIMB LEADS: PRECORDIAL LEADS:
P
QRS
S-T

INTERPRETATION, SERIAL CHANGES, IMPLICATIONS:

PATIENT'S IDENTIFICATION   INTERPRETED BY
Robert Booth   M.D.
#8-6012780   ECG NO.   WARD   R.M.
                        DATE

4.10 Equipment Maintenance

Care and maintenance of the ECG machine must be done and is your responsibility. Become familiar with the manufacturer's instructions for operation and maintenance of the ECG machine. The operator's manual for the machine you are using will include specific directions about routine care and maintenance. General day-to-day care and maintenance include cleaning the ECG machine and stocking the supplies, such as electrodes, skin preparation, paper, and cleaning supplies.

Maintaining the ECG Equipment

Cleaning the ECG machine and maintaining the supplies are necessary for safe and efficient ECG recording and accurate tracings.

Keep the ECG machine clean to prevent transmission of infection and to create a positive image of yourself and the facility where you are employed. Use a small amount of nonabrasive cleaner on the equipment case, cover, and control panel. Wipe the machine dry with a soft cloth. Follow the specific directions in the operator's manual for the disinfection procedure.

The cables and reusable electrodes should be disinfected frequently. Use a soft cloth moistened with disinfectant and wipe the entire cable and reusable electrode. You can also use packaged disinfectant wipes if they are available. Keep these available on the ECG cart. Do not place the cables or ECG machine in fluid or use heat sterilization. Do not use acetone, ether, or other harsh chemicals or solvents. Always follow the manufacturer's directions for best results.

Reusable electrodes require additional attention. After each use, the electrodes must be cleaned to prevent a buildup of gel or paste. Scour them once a week with an abrasive kitchen cleanser to prevent corrosion and restore the bright finish to the contact surfaces. Do not forget to clean the metal tips of the patient cable. Electrolyte gel or paste can build up on the metal tips and prevent proper contact with the electrodes. The electrode straps should be washed and checked for cracks. Replace any broken or cracked straps immediately.

When using disposable electrodes, carefully maintain the alligator clips used for attachment. Check them to ensure that the pins fit snugly on the electrode. Check for small amounts of electrolyte paste or gel that may cling to the clips. These bits of paste may prevent good contact with the electrodes (see Figure 4-10).

Wipe down the patient cables and lead wires with a damp cloth. Replace them neatly on the ECG machine for storage (see Figure 4-11). Inspect them regularly for cracks or fraying. Replace any cables that are damaged.

Checkpoint Question 4-10

1. Why should you know how to troubleshoot and maintain the equipment for an ECG?

_____

_____

Answer the preceding question and complete the "Equipment Maintenance" activity on the student CD under Chapter 4 before you proceed to the next section.

Figure 4-10 This alligator type clip is frequently used for the ECG. Wipe these clips clean after use to prevent electrolyte gel or paste from getting stuck between the teeth of the clip.

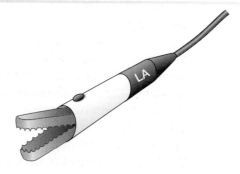

Figure 4-11 Before storing clean each lead wire and clip with disinfectant. For safety, inspect each wire for cracks or fraying.

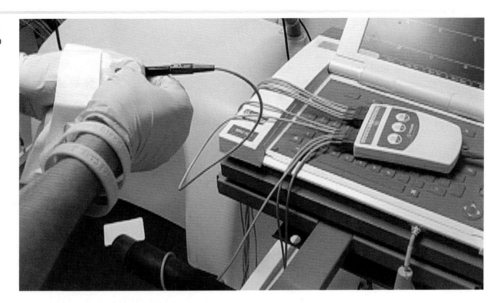

4.11 Pediatric ECG

When preparing a child for an ECG, it is important to give simple directions that he or she can understand. Identify yourself and explain what you are going to do. Allow the child to ask questions. Avoid technical words like *electrodes* and *electrocardiogram*. Use the word "stickers" to describe electrodes. If the child is fearful of the "stickers," allow them to place the stickers on a toy, doll, or parent. This will show the child that the procedure does not hurt. Explain that you are going to take a "picture" of the child's heart. Because children can usually identify with picture taking, this will help them understand that they need to be still during the "picture."

Always identify the child by name and check his or her identification armband. If the parents are present, you may allow them to stay. For a small child or infant, the parent can assist by letting the child lie quietly in his or her arms. A fussy infant may be soothed by using a pacifier. If you are unable to soothe an irritable infant, you may need to wait until he or she falls asleep. For older children, you can allow them to apply their own arm and leg electrodes. Adolescents may prefer to be alone with you during the procedure. Ask them if they would like their parent(s) to stay or leave.

When the ECG tracing is completed, talk about the procedure. Give verbal praise and be supportive. Reward the child with an age-appropriate item or activity such as stickers or a special trip to the playroom.

Smaller electrodes should be used for pediatric patients. Special smaller electrodes are available and may be used. In addition, frequently you will need to adjust the paper speed to 50 mm/sec for infants or children with very fast heart rates. This will allow the physician to view each of the deflections on the ECG tracing. If you make this adjustment, it must be noted on the ECG recording when completed.

An ECG for a child is performed with the same lead placement as for an adult. The chest lead V6 must be placed exactly on the midaxillary line. Because of the small size of the chest, correct placement becomes even more important. Small differences in placement can make a difference in the ECG tracing. Because of crowding on the chest, it may be necessary to move the V3 lead to the right side of the chest. It should be placed on the right side in the same location as it normally would be on the left. This is known as a V3 right (V3R) (see Figure 4-12).

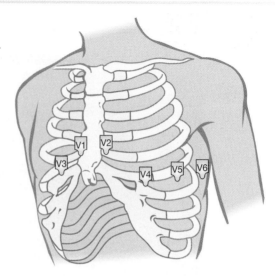

Figure 4-12 For infants and small children, you may need to place V3 on the right side of the chest to prevent crowding of the chest electrodes. This alternate method of placement is known as V3R and is sometimes used on adults.

Checkpoint Questions 4-11

1. Why do you frequently need to adjust the paper speed to 50 mm/sec for infants and small children?

_____

_____

2. When you change the paper speed to 50 mm/sec, what should you do?

_____

_____

 Answer the preceding questions and complete the "Pediatric ECG" activity on the student CD under Chapter 4 before you proceed to the next section.

4.12 Special Patient Considerations

Occasionally you will need to record lead tracings other than the basic 12. You may need to record a heart rhythm strip, which is a single strip showing only one lead tracing. The heart rhythm is usually produced in lead II and is about 10 seconds of running time. Many ECG machines will print this strip on the bottom of the 12-lead tracing or following the completion of the 12-lead recording. A rhythm strip will be used to check for heart rhythm abnormalities. You may also be asked to provide a V4R on an adult for cases of right ventricular infarction.

You may encounter other circumstances that require you to make modifications to the basic 12-lead procedure. When changes in the placement of leads is necessary for any reason, a note should be included on the tracing. Consider the following when placing leads and recording tracings in a patient's chart:

- V1 and V2 may have to be placed higher due to breast implants.
- Do not place the electrode on a woman's breast. Move the breast with the back of your hand and place the electrode under it. If this is done, note on the ECG tracing that the electrodes (V3, V4, and V5) are placed lower than required.
- If a woman has had a mastectomy, note this on the ECG tracing. It may alter the ECG results.

Figure 4-13 Use these lead placements for patients with dextrocardia, a condition in which the left ventricle, left atrium, aortic arch, and stomach are located on the right side of the chest.

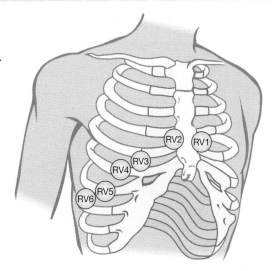

- If the patient is an amputee, place the limb leads on the upper chest and lower abdomen instead of on the arms and legs. Make sure the leads are in the same place on each side of the body.
- A pregnant woman should have the lower limb leads placed on the thighs, not the abdomen. Place the patient on her left side slightly, by using a small rolled towel under the right hip to reduce pressure on the inferior vena cava. Document on the ECG that the patient is pregnant and the number of months.
- Geriatric patients generally have thin skin, which is part of the normal aging process. Apply the electrodes carefully and remove gently to prevent damage to their skin. Geriatric patients may have some readings on the ECG tracing that are age-related and are considered normal.
- If the patient is unable to lie on his or her back, be sure to indicate on the tracing the position of the patient during the tracing.
- When someone is in a permanent fetal position with arms drawn tightly over his or her chest, you may need to place the electrodes on the back. They will need to be positioned over the heart on the left side of the back. Today's small, thin, disposable electrodes are easier to place under a patient's arms, so place on the back only if necessary.
- A condition that would require the changing of lead placement is **dextrocardia,** when the organs in the chest are on the opposite or right side of the chest. The leads should be reversed (mirror image) from the usual lead placement. This is the only case where the aVR tracing will produce a positive deflection. On the ECG tracing report, you should indicate that you did a right-side ECG (see Figure 4-13).

You may be asked to perform a 15- or 18-lead ECG as ordered by the physician. These expanded data tracings enable the physician to be able to detect problems with the right ventricular and posterior wall of the left ventricle. The National Heart Attack Alert Program recommends the use of these nonstandard ECGs to increase the awareness and detection of heart attacks in these areas. These leads are commonly identified as right precordial leads (V4R, V5R, V6R) and posterior leads (V7, V8, V9). When these leads are combined with the 12 leads, you obtain the 15- or 18-lead combination.

Some facilities will have specialized equipment, but it is not essential. You can obtain the ECG tracing by adding these leads with the standard 12-lead ECG machine. This procedure can be simple when knowing where to place the electrodes. First, run a standard 12-lead ECG as described earlier. Secondly, you will use the precordial leads (V1 to V6), place additional electrodes in the appropriate locations, and run a second 12-lead ECG. It is important that you do not forget to write on the labels of the new leads, especially when using a three-channel ECG machine. The patient must lie as still as possible to avoid artifact, which can occur in the back leads. The right side of the chest leads are located as follows:

- V4R is located at the right midclavicular line in the fifth intercostal space; reposition the V3 lead to this location.
- V5R is located at the right anterior axillary line in a straight line from V4R; you will reposition the V2 lead to this location.
- V6R is located at the right midaxillary line in a straight line from the V5R; you will move the V1 lead to this location.

The posterior leads (or leads on the patient's back) are focusing on the posterior aspect of the heart:

- V7 is located at the left **posterior axillary line** (an imaginary line on the back of the chest that runs vertically from the shoulder down on the outer edge of the rib cage) in a straight line from V6; you will reposition the V4 lead to this location.
- V8 is located at the **midscapular line** (an imaginary line on the back of the chest that runs vertically through the center of the scapula) in a straight line from V7; you will reposition the V5 lead to this location.

Figure 4-14 For a 15- or 18-lead ECG, the chest leads are commonly identified as right precordial leads (V4R, V5R, V6R) and posterior leads (V7, V8, V9).

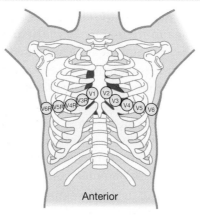
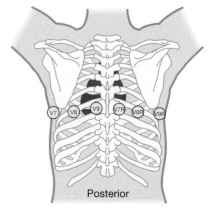

Anterior

Posterior

V1 — Fourth intercostal space at the right sternal border, right chest

V2 — Fourth intercostal space at the left sternal border, left chest

V3 — Midway between locations V2 and V4, left chest

V4 — Midclavicular line in the fifth intercostal space, left chest

V5 — Anterior axillary line on the same horizontal level as V4, left chest

V6 — Midaxillary line on the same horizontal level as V4 and V5, left chest

V3R — Midway between locations V1 and V4R, right chest

V4R — Midclavicular line in the fifth intercostal space, right chest

V5R — Anterior axillary line on the same horizontal level as V4R. right chest

V6R — Midaxillary line on the same horizontal level as V4R and V5R, right chest

V7R — Right posterior axillary line, V6R level

V8R — Under right midscapular line, V6R level

V9R — Right paraspinal border, V6R level

V7 — Left posterior axillary line, V6 level

V8 — Under left midscapular line, V6 level

V9 — Left paraspinal border, V6 level

- V9 is located at **paraspinal line** (an imaginary line on the spine that runs vertically through the side of the spine) in a straight line from the V8 lead; you will move the V6 lead to this location. (see Figure 4-14).

When you record a 15-lead or 18-lead ECG tracing, it is critical that you indicate a modification in the ECG tracing because the electrodes are focused on a different aspect of the heart and could potentially provide the wrong information if not noted.

Checkpoint Question 4-12

1. What should you remember when asked to record a 15-lead or 18-lead ECG?

_____

_____

 Answer the preceding question and complete the "Special Patient Considerations" activity on the student CD under Chapter 4 before you proceed to the next section.

4.13 Handling Emergencies

Cardiac or Respiratory Arrest

During a cardiac or respiratory arrest, frequentcy called a Code Blue emergency, be ready to perform the tracing as quickly and efficiently as possible. An ECG is usually ordered "stat" in these situations. If possible, enter the patient's information into the ECG machine. Remain available but out of the way until the ECG is needed. You may need to take just the machine into the room and not the cart, if space is limited.

Because the patient's condition changes frequently during a Code Blue emergency, you may need to perform two ECGs in a row. Perform the first ECG and leave the electrodes in place in order to perform the second ECG quickly. Indicate on the tracing "repeat ECG—same lead placement." This will make the physician aware that the electrodes were not removed in between tracings.

Seizure

If a patient has a **seizure** during the ECG, stay with him or her. Protect the patient from injury. Do not try to restrain the patient. Call for help and report the seizure. Once the seizure is over, perform the ECG again and write on the ECG strip "postseizure."

Checkpoint Question 4-13

1. What should you do if your patient has a seizure while you are starting to record an ECG?

_____

_____

 Answer the preceding question above and complete the "Handling Emergencies" activity on the student CD under Chapter 4 before you proceed to the next section.

Chapter Summary

- The patient, the room, and the equipment must be properly prepared prior to performing an ECG.
- When a patient refuses an ECG, you should identify the cause, alleviate any fears, notify your supervisor, and document the refusal on the medical record.
- In order to place the electrodes properly for an ECG you must be able to locate anatomical landmarks including the midclavicular line, anterior axillary line, intercostal spaces, suprasternal notch, and the angle of Louis.
- Following standard precautions and performing hand hygiene are two ways to prevent infection during an ECG. In addition, isolation precautions may be used in a hospital or other in-patient health care facility.
- Maintain safety during an ECG by checking the plug and power cord, raising the bed to a working height, keeping the side rail up on the opposite side of the bed, and performing hand hygiene and wearing personal protective equipment, when necessary.
- To ensure HIPAA compliance when identifying a patient, you must use at least two patient identifiers, neither of which should be the patient's room number.
- Three types of artifact include somatic tremor caused by muscle movement, wandering baseline usually caused by improperly applied electrodes, or poor skin prep, and AC interference caused by some type of electrical interference.
- ECGs are recorded electronically and in paper fashion. Although they may be "read" by the machine, they must be provided promptly in a proper format to the practitioner who will be interpreting them.
- Single channel ECG tracings are cut and mounted for easy viewing and interpretation.
- During a pediatric ECG the chest lead V3 may need to be placed on the right side of the chest due to the small size of the chest.
- Many special patient considerations can occur during an ECG, such as for female patients, pregnant patients, amputees, and geriatric patients.
- Upon completion of an ECG the equipment must be cleaned and stored properly according to your facility guidelines and the manufacturer's recommendations.

Chapter Review

Matching I

Match the landmark with its location. Place the letter on the corresponding line.

_____ **1.** suprasternal notch

_____ **2.** fifth intercostal space

_____ **3.** manubrium

_____ **4.** right clavicle

a. extends from the sternum to the scapula

b. the space between the fifth and sixth ribs

c. the top of the sternum

d. the dip at the base of the neck just above where the clavicle attaches to the sternum

Match the lead to its correct placement. Place the letter on the corresponding line.

_____ **5.** V1

_____ **6.** V2

_____ **7.** V3

_____ **8.** V4

_____ **9.** V5

_____ **10.** V6

a. fifth intercostal space, at the anterior axillary line

b. fourth intercostal space, left sternal border

c. fifth intercostal space, at the midaxillary line

d. fifth intercostal space at the midclavicular line

e. fourth intercostal space, right sternal border

f. halfway between V2 and V4

Match the imaginary line with its location. Place the letter on the corresponding line.

_____ **11.** midclavicular line

_____ **12.** midaxillary line

_____ **13.** anterior axillary line

a. front of the axilla

b. middle of the axilla

c. usually passes through the nipple line

Multiple Choice

Circle the correct answer.

14. For placement of the electrodes, how is the ICS located?
    a. Locating the sternum and feeling for a dip at the edge
    b. Finding the ribs near the nipple line
    c. Locating the clavicle and feeling for a dent directly below it
    d. Locating the space between the clavicle and V4

15. What would be the first and most appropriate thing to say if a patient refuses an ECG?
    a. "Maybe you can tell me why you don't wish to have an ECG done."
    b. "Don't worry; it only takes a few seconds."
    c. "Your doctor has ordered this test and it must be done."
    d. "I will have to report you to my supervisor immediately."

16. When applying chest leads, V4 is placed
    a. midway between V3 and V5.
    b. at the fourth ICS, right sternal border.
    c. at the fifth ICS, left midclavicular line.
    d. at the fourth ICS, left sternal border.

17. When applying chest leads, V2 is placed
    a. midway between V3 and V5.
    b. at the fourth ICS, right sternal border.
    c. at the fifth ICS, left midclavicular line.
    d. at the fourth ICS, left sternal border.

18. To prevent disease transmission during an ECG, you should
    a. Check the ground prong.
    b. Wash your hands.
    c. Raise the side rail.
    d. Lower the bed.

19. Safety procedures specific to the ECG include the following:
    a. Wash hands, clean up all spills immediately.
    b. Lower bed, raise the side rail.
    c. Check the ground prong, give the call signal.
    d. Check the lead wires, insulation, and ground prong.

20. Which of the following would *not* be done prior to performing an ECG?
    a. Receive and validate the order.
    b. Clean the leads and write ECG variations on tracing.
    c. Check and change paper if necessary.
    d. Enter patient data into machine.

21. When applying chest leads, V1 is placed
    a. midway between V3 and V5.
    b. at the fourth ICS, right sternal border.
    c. at the fifth ICS, left midclavicular line.
    d. at the fourth ICS, left sternal border.

22. Marks on the ECG tracing caused by another source of activity are
    a. asystole.
    b. conduction marks.
    c. artifacts.
    d. wandering baseline.

23. Somatic tremors are caused by
    a. electrical current leak.
    b. tracing drifts away from center.
    c. muscle movement.
    d. contact with another electrical device.

24. You noticed a wandering baseling on the ECG tracing. What measure(s) should you do to correct the problem?
    a. Apply new electrodes.
    b. Reposition the electrodes.
    c. Ensure that the wires are not crossing.
    d. All of the above.

25. You notice that leads I and II have a lot of artifact while recording the 12 lead. Which electrode is probably not placed appropriately?
    a. Right arm
    b. Left arm
    c. Left leg
    d. None of the above

26. Which of the following is *not* a specific type of isolation precaution implemented for hospitalized patients?
    a. AIDS precautions
    b. Droplet precautions
    c. Airborne precautions
    d. Contact precautions

27. Which of the following are ways to correct AC interference?
    a. Unplug electrical equipment, move bed away from wall.
    b. Apply electrodes securely, remove tension from lead wires.
    c. Have patient place hands under his or her buttocks, remind patient not to move.
    d. Replace loose electrodes and have the patient turn slightly to the side.

28. Which of the following are ways to correct somatic tremor?
    a. Unplug electrical equipment, move bed away from wall.
    b. Apply electrodes securely, remove tension from lead wires.
    c. Have patient place hands under his or her buttocks, remind patient not to move.
    d. Replace loose electrodes and have the patient turn slightly to the side.

29. Which of the following are ways to correct wandering baseline?
    a. Unplug electrical equipment, move bed away from wall.
    b. Apply electrodes securely, remove tension from lead wires.
    c. Have patient place hands under his or her buttocks, remind patient not to move.
    d. Replace loose electrodes and have the patient turn slightly to the side.

30. When applying chest leads, V6 is placed
    a. in line with V4 on the midaxillary line.
    b. at the fourth ICS, right sternal border.
    c. at the fifth ICS, left midclavicular line.
    d. at the fourth ICS, left sternal border.

31. If your patient has an amputated left lower leg, you should place the electrodes as follows:
    a. LL on left upper leg, RL on right lower leg
    b. LL on left lower abdomen, RL on right lower abdomen
    c. LL on left lower leg, RL on right upper leg
    d. LL on left lower abdomen, RL on right lower leg

32. When performing a 12-lead ECG on an infant or small child, do all of the following *except*
    a. Speak in children's terms.
    b. Use smaller ECG electrodes.
    c. Perform a V3R tracing.
    d. Use a special ECG machine.

33. Approach the patient from the _____ when performing an ECG.
    a. left side
    b. right side
    c. top
    d. bottom

True/False

Read each statement and determine if it is true or false. Circle the T or F. For false (F) statements, correct them to "make them true" on the lines provided.

T   F   **34.** Natural skin oils, moisturizers, and perspiration can contribute to artifact on an ECG tracing. _____

_____

T   F   **35.** The letter *R* is placed after any tracing when the electrode has been placed on the right side of the patient's chest. _____

_____

T   F   **36.** Because an ECG is *not* an invasive procedure, it is not necessary to wear personal protective equipment (PPE) when performing this procedure under any circumstances.

_____

_____

Matching II

_____ **37.** intercostal space (ICS)

_____ **38.** midaxillary line

_____ **39.** stat

_____ **40.** anterior axillary line

_____ **41.** artifact

_____ **42.** seizure

_____ **43.** midclavicular line

_____ **44.** somatic tremor

_____ **45.** angle of Louis

_____ **46.** AC Interference

_____ **47.** wandering baseline

_____ **48.** sternal border

_____ **49.** dextrocardia

_____ **50.** midscapular line

a. an interruption of the electrical activity of the brain that causes involuntary muscle movement and sometimes unconsciousness

b. a boney prominence located approximately 1 inch below the suprasternal notch, where the manubrium and the body of the sternum are joined

c. outer edge of the sternum

d. the space between two ribs

e. an imaginary line on the chest that runs vertically through the center of the clavicle

f. when the tracing of an ECG drifts away from the center of the paper; also called baseline shift (It has many causes, which can be corrected.)

g. an imaginary vertical line that starts in the middle of the axillary region (armpit)

h. unwanted marks on the ECG caused by electrical activity from sources other than the heart

i. unwanted markings on the ECG tracing caused by other electrical sources

j. an imaginary vertical line on the back that starts in the middle of the scapula

k. immediately

l. voluntary or involuntary muscle movement; also known as body tremor

m. an imaginary vertical line starting at the edge of the chest where the axillary region begins

n. when the organs of the chest are on the reverse side

51. (1.–9.) Identify the landmarks on the chest drawing. Label each line.

1. _____

2. _____

3. _____

4. _____

5. _____

6. _____

7. _____

8. _____

9. _____

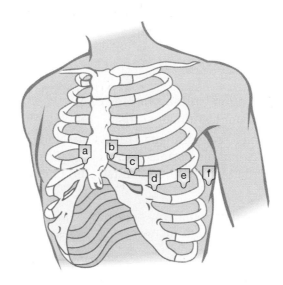

52. Identify each lead and describe its location for a 12-lead ECG.

a. _____

b. _____

c. _____

d. _____

e. _____

f. _____

What Should You Do? *Critical Thinking Application*

Read the following situations and use your critical thinking skills to determine how you would handle each. Write your answer in detail in the space provided.

53. You are working in a local hospital and are called to perform an ECG on a patient who is in a coma and was admitted to the hospital because of a myocardial infarction. You set up the machine and begin to run the ECG and the tracing is a flat line. You know that a flat line is serious. What would be the first thing you do?

   _____

   _____

54. Your patient has Parkinson's disease. During the procedure, you notice a lot of artifact. What kind of artifact would you expect it to be? How could you reduce the artifact?

   _____

   _____

55. You are performing an ECG on a patient and he or she begins to complain of chest pain. What should you do?

   _____

   _____

56. When you finish performing an ECG, the patient asks you for a copy. What do you do?

   _____

   _____

Get Connected *Internet Activity*

Visit the McGraw-Hill Higher Education Online Learning Center *Electrocardiography for Health Care Personnel* Web site at **www.mhhe.com/healthcareskills** to complete the following activity.

15-and 18-lead ECG The American Association of Critical Care Nurses describes the steps and lead placement for obtaining more than the normal 12-lead ECG. Search their Web site or use a search engine to find information that will help you understand the rationale and placement of the electrodes.

When using a search engine ensure that you always look at the source of your information. Medical centers, professional organizations, and manufacturers' Web sites are more reliable and will provide you with accurate information.

Using the Student CD

Now that you have completed the material in the chapter text, return to the student CD and complete any chapter activities you have not yet done. Practice your terminology with the "Key Term Concentration" game. Review the chapter material with the "Spin the Wheel" game. Take the final chapter test and complete the troubleshooting question and email or print your results to document your proficiency for this chapter

ECG Interpretation and Clinical Significance

5

Learning Outcomes

- Summarize the process of evaluating ECG tracings and determining the presence of dysrhythmias.
- Identify the criteria used for classification of the dysrhythmias including rhythm, rate, P wave configuration, PR interval measurement, and QRS duration measurement.
- Describe the various rhythms and dysrhythmias including sinus, atrial, junctional, supraventricular, heart block, bundle branch block, ventricular, and pacemaker.
- Identify the dysrhythmias using the criteria for classification.
- Explain how each dysrhythmia may affect the patient.
- Discuss basic patient care and treatment for dysrhythmias.
- Describe an electronic pacemaker, its function, and the normal pacemaker rhythm characteristics.
- Identify the steps in evaluating electronic pacemaker function on an ECG tracing.

Key Terms

apnea	bigeminy
asystole	biphasic
atrial kick	blocked or nonconducted
automaticity	impulse

bradycardia	neurological
bundle branch block	oversensing
capture	pacemaker competition
cardiac output parameters	pacemaker malfunctioning
electronic pacemaker	palpitations
focus (pl. foci)	quadgeminy
hypotension	supraventricular
inhibited	syncope
ischemia	tachycardia
J point	trigeminy
loss of capture	triggered
malsensing	vagal tone

5.1 Introduction

As discussed in Chapter 1, the ECG is an important tool used for the diagnosis and treatment of various cardiac and other related diseases. The recorded tracing of the ECG waveforms produced by the heart can tell you basic information about a patient's condition. The ability to evaluate various ECG waveforms is an important skill for many health care professionals including nurses, doctors, and medical assistants. In addition, as a multiskilled health care employee you may be required to determine if an ECG is normal or abnormal and be able to respond to a cardiac emergency, if necessary. You will follow your scope of practice and the policy at your place of employment when evaluating and reporting dysrhythmias.

As you have already learned, the ECG waveform has various components such as waves, segments, and intervals that are evaluated and classified based on their size, length of time, and location on the tracing. All of these different components determine the type of cardiac rhythm. In order to evaluate a rhythm, you must first understand each component and its normal appearance. When these components differ from the expected norm, a dysrhythmia (or arrhythmia) is indicated. Remember, an abnormal ECG tracing may only be the result of artifact. The tracing must be evaluated for artifact prior to the evaluation of the heart rhythm.

The process of determining or labeling the type of cardiac dysrhythmia can be challenging. The best approach in determining the actual rhythm is to take on the role of a detective. Detectives will gather all the information they can before determining who is the suspect or how something has happened. The process of ECG analysis is similar. We first gather all the data regarding the different waveforms and their patterns. The next step is to match all the information to the specific ECG rhythm criteria in order to classify the various cardiac dysrhythmias.

In this chapter, you are introduced to the rhythm criteria used to identify the various cardiac dysrhythmias. You will learn the process of evaluating dysrhythmia, which will lay a strong foundation for your beginning practice or continued education in electrocardiography. Most importantly, after completing this chapter you should be able to recognize abnormalities in the cardiac rhythm and respond appropriately.

1. What is evaluated and classified when determining dysrhythmias?

_____

_____

5.2 Identifying the Components of the Rhythm

ECG analysis consists of a five-step process of gathering data about each rhythm strip. These steps include evaluating the following components of the ECG rhythm strips:

- Rhythm (regularity)
- Rate
- P wave configuration
- PR interval
- QRS duration and configuration

Once the information is gathered, the data are compared to the specific criteria for each dysrhythmia. Cardiac dysrhythmia interpretation is an art. Frequently, you will find practitioners discussing how to classify a dysrhythmia because patients may experience a variety of different cardiac dysrhythmias at the same time. This makes it difficult to determine the origin of the dysrhythmia or to classify it. The more interpretation you perform, the more efficient you become in classifying the rhythm.

Before you begin the steps, you should know that lead II is the most common monitoring lead. It is used in this chapter unless otherwise specified.

Step 1: Determining the ECG Rhythm or Regularity

Determining the rhythm involves evaluating the pattern of how the atria and ventricles contract. The rhythm can occur in regular or irregular intervals. Each chamber of the heart is assessed for its type of pattern. In Chapter 3, you learned that the P wave represents atrial contraction and the QRS complex represents ventricular contraction. The rhythm of atrial contraction is evaluated by assessing the regularity or irregularity of the occurrence of the P waves. The QRS complexes are assessed to evaluate ventricular contraction. Calipers are used for this portion of the analysis to measure the distance between the P waves and the width of the QRS complex (see Figure 5-1).

The P-P wave interval should be evaluated first. The caliper interval is established when the first point of the caliper is placed on the beginning of one P wave and the second point on the beginning of the next P wave. Measuring several of these intervals determines if the P waves are occurring in a regular sequence. At least 10 seconds of the ECG tracing of P waves are measured to determine if the P waves occur in a regular or irregular rhythm throughout the rhythm strip (see Figure 5-2).

Next, determine the rhythm of the QRS complex. Since the QRS complex is a configuration of three possible waveforms, it is important to analyze this interval from the same waveform in each of the QRS complexes. For

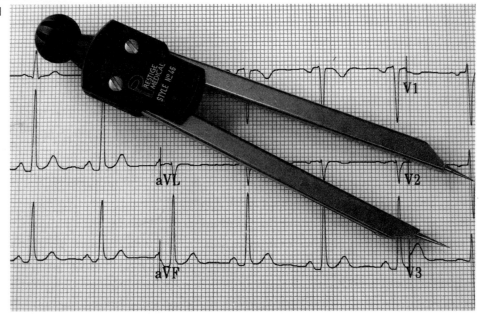

Figure 5-1 Calipers are used to measure ECG tracing.

example, it is often easier to see the R wave of the QRS complex. Measuring the R-R wave interval is easy due to its upward deflection (see Figure 5-3). Occasionally, the QRS complex does not exhibit an R wave, in which case you can use the point of the Q and S wave junction as an easy point of evaluation. Most importantly, you must measure the same part of the waveform for each QRS complex to determine the regularity of the ventricular depolarization. The first point of the caliper should be placed on the first QRS complex and the other point placed on the next QRS complex. The interval should be evaluated throughout at least a 6-second strip to determine the rhythm of the QRS complexes.

Step 2: Determining the Atrial and Ventricular Rate

The method used to calculate the heart rate is based on whether the rhythm is regular or irregular. The heart rate must be determined for both atria and ventricles. The atrial rate is determined by the P-P wave interval measurements, and the ventricular rate is determined by the R-R wave measurement. Most frequently, the atrial and ventricular rates will be the same; sometimes, however, the rates may be different due to conditions occurring in the myocardium. It is important to note if the atrial rate is different from the ventricular rate since this will help narrow the selection of dysrhythmias. The methods used to differentiate the rates are described in the following sections.

Regular Rhythm

Once you have determined that the rhythm is regular, you can use this method to calculate the atrial and ventricular rate. The caliper interval of the P-P or R-R measurement is placed on the ECG paper to determine the number of small boxes or duration of time. (Remember from Chapter 3 that each small box is equal to 0.04 seconds.) Move the caliper interval to the top or the bottom of the page so that the number of boxes can be determined without interference from the ECG tracing. Once you have counted the small boxes,

Figure 5-2 Measuring the
P-to-P wave interval.

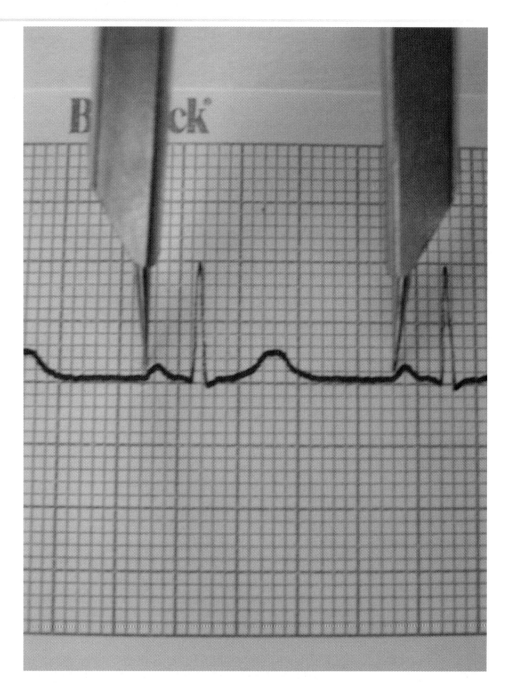

divide the number into 1500 to calculate the heart rate. The ventricular rate
is determined in the same manner except you will need to count the number of boxes *between* the QRS complexes. Table 5-1 provides the heart rates
based on the number of small boxes between the two P or two R waves. This
method of calculation provides an accurate heart rate similar to measuring
a person's pulse, unlike the method described in Chapter 3, which provides
only an estimate. The actual rate is extremely important when the heart rate
is either **tachycardia** (more than 100 beats per minute) or **bradycardia** (less
than 60 beats per minute).

Irregular Rhythm

When the rhythm is irregular, as determined in Step 1, the interval between
the P waves or the QRS complexes is not constant. To determine the heart rate

Figure 5-3 Computerized caliper measurement of the R-to-R wave interval.

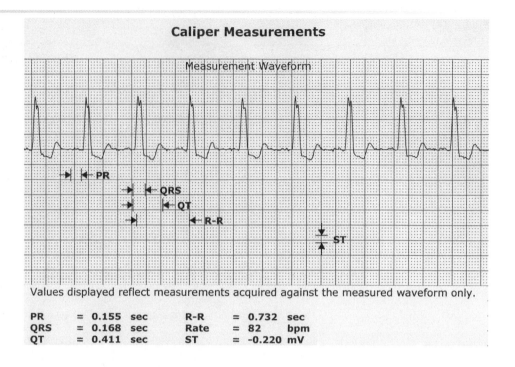

Caliper Measurements

Measurement Waveform

Values displayed reflect measurements acquired against the measured waveform only.

PR	= 0.155 sec	R-R	= 0.732 sec
QRS	= 0.168 sec	Rate	= 82 bpm
QT	= 0.411 sec	ST	= -0.220 mV

for an irregular rhythm, use the 6-second method as described in Chapter 3. Simply multiply the number of P waves and QRS complexes in a 6-second strip by 10. This method is often used in emergencies to determine an estimated heart rate (pulse rate) for the patient.

Step 3: Identifying the P Wave Configuration

Analyzing P waves and their relationship with the QRS complex is necessary to determine the type of dysrhythmia. The P wave reflects the atrial contraction and how the electrical current is moving through the atria. The relationship between the P wave and QRS complex provides information regarding the coordination between atrial and ventricular contractions. Several questions need to be answered when analyzing the P wave.

- *Are the shapes and waveforms all the same?* If they appear to be different, the route in which the current is moving through the atria is not on the same pathway. Sometimes the P wave may not exist.
- *Does each P wave have a QRS complex following it?* In normal conduction pathways, the QRS complex always follows the P wave. If there are additional P waves or QRS complexes present without a P wave in front, the normal conduction pathway may not have been used and the atria and ventricles are not contracting together.

Step 4: Measuring the PR Interval

The PR interval measures the length of time it takes the electrical current to be initiated at the sinoatrial node and travel through the electrical current pathway to cause a ventricular contraction. The PR interval is determined by measuring from the beginning of the P wave, or its up slope, to the beginning of the QRS complex. This is the first indication of ventricular depolarization. Not all tracings will show a Q wave. In the absense of a Q wave, the second caliper tip is placed at the beginning of the R wave. (Please review

TABLE 5-1 Calculating Heart Rates with a Regular Rhythm

Small Boxes in P-P or R-R Interval	Heart Rate	Small Boxes in P-P or R-R Interval	Heart Rate	Small Boxes in P-P or R-R Interval	Heart Rate
4	375	20	75	36	42
5	300	21	71	37	40
6	250	22	68	38	39
7	214	23	65	39	38
8	188	24	62	40	38
9	167	25	60	41	37
10	150	26	58	42	36
11	136	27	55	43	35
12	125	28	54	44	34
13	115	29	52	45	33
14	107	30	50	46	33
15	100	31	48	47	32
16	94	32	47	48	31
17	88	33	45	49	31
18	83	34	44	50	30
19	79	35	43		

A rate calculator can also be used for regular rhythms. The start mark is placed at the first P wave or R wave, whichever you are using. Where the next consecutive P or R wave lines up is the approximate heart rate. See the following figure.

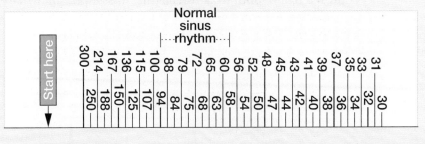

Figure 2-10 if necessary.) The normal range of the PR interval is 0.12 to 0.20 second (see Figure 5-4).

When determining the measurements, the time interval should always be in multiples of 0.02 second, which represents one-half of the smallest box. To effectively determine measurements to 0.01 second, the small box on the ECG paper would need to be divided into four smaller divisions. ***This can be done effectively only with a computer, not a practitioner's eyes.***

Figure 5-4 The PR interval measured from the beginning of the P wave to the first indication of ventricular depolarization which is usually the beginning of the QRS complex.

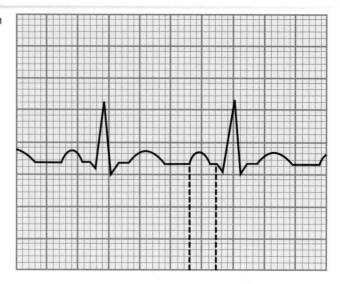

PR intervals are also evaluated to ensure that the measurements are the same from one PR interval to the next. If the intervals have different measurements, either the electrical current is being delayed for some reason or it may be initiating from locations other than the sinoatrial node.

Step 5: Measuring the QRS Duration and Analyzing the Configuration

Measuring the QRS complex is essential in determining the duration of time it takes for the ventricles to depolarize or contract. This information is helpful in discriminating between different dysrhythmias. If the QRS complex is narrow, or within the normal limits of 0.06 to 0.10 second, current has traveled through the normal ventricular conduction pathways to activate the ventricles to contract. When the QRS complex is wide, 0.12 second or greater, the current is taking longer than normal to contract the ventricles.

To measure the QRS duration and configuration, place the first caliper point where the QRS complex starts and the second point at the **J point** (see Figure 5-5). The J point is located where the S wave stops and the ST segment is initiated. It marks the point at which ventricular depolarization is completed and repolarization begins. It is important to carefully identify this

Figure 5-5 The J point is where the S wave stops and the ST segment is initiated.

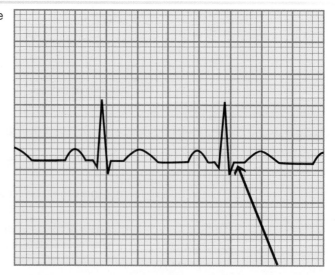

Figure 5-6 Measure the QRS duration from the beginning of the QRS complex to the J point.

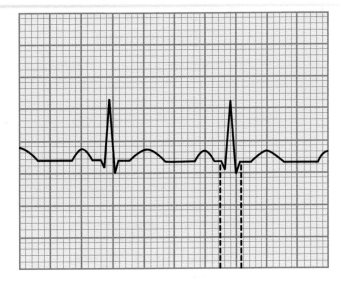

ending point of the QRS complex, since many times the ST segment may not be at the isoelectric line.

Several questions need to be answered when determining the QRS measurement and configuration (see Figure 5-6).

- Are all the QRS complexes of equal length?
- What is the actual measurement, and is it within the normal limits?
- Do all QRS complexes look alike, and are the unusual QRS complexes associated with an ectopic beat?

After you have completed these five steps of identifying the components of the rhythm, you will then compare the information to the specific criteria for classifying each of the dysrhythmias. The rest of this chapter explains the specific criteria for classification related to common rhythms and dysrhythmias that will help you identify the various ECG rhythms.

Checkpoint Questions 5-2

1. Name the five components that must be evaluated on a rhythm strip.

   _____

   _____

2. A regular rhythm has 19 small boxes between the P-P interval. What is the heart rate?

   _____

   _____

3. After you measure the QRS duration and configuration, what other questions need to be answered?

   _____

   _____

 Answer the preceding questions and complete the "Identifying the Components of the Rhythm" activity on the student CD under Chapter 5 before you proceed to the next section.

5.3 Rhythms Originating from the Sinus Node (Sinus Beat)

The sinoatrial node is the normal or "primary" pacemaker of the heart. It generates an electrical impulse that travels through the normal conduction pathway to cause the myocardium to depolarize. Electrical current starts at the sinoatrial node and travels the normal conduction pathway to the atrioventrical node and continues through the bundle of His and bundle branches to the ventricles. Because the rhythm starts at the sinoatrial node, it is called sinus rhythm. The electrical current is produced at the sinus node at a rate of 60 to 100 beats per minute. The rates of the rhythm will vary, and the types of sinus beats may include sinus rhythm, sinus bradycardia, sinus tachycardia, and sinus dysrhythmia.

Normal Sinus Rhythm

Sinus rhythm is reflective of a normally functioning conduction system. The electrical current is following the normal conduction pathway without interference from other bodily systems or disease processes (see Figure 5-7).

Criteria for Classification

- *Rhythm:* The intervals between the two P and two R waves will occur in a consistent pattern.
- *Rate:* Both the atrial and ventricular rate will be between 60 and 100 beats.
- *P wave configuration:* The P waves will have the same shape and are usually upright in deflection on the rhythm strip. A P wave will appear in front of every QRS complex.
- *PR interval:* The PR interval measurement will be between 0.12 and 0.20 second, which is within normal limits. Each PR interval will be the same, without any variations.
- *QRS duration and configuration:* The QRS duration and configuration measurement will be between 0.06 and 0.10 second, which is within normal limits. Each QRS duration and configuration will be without any variations from PQRST complex to complex.

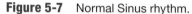

What's Unique about Normal Sinus Rhythm?

Sinus rhythm is the only rhythm for which all five steps are within normal limits.

Figure 5-7 Normal Sinus rhythm.

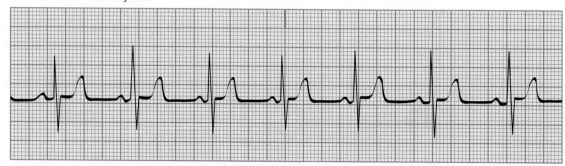

TABLE 5-2 Signs and Symptoms of Decreased Cardiac Output

Observe for any of these signs and symptoms associated with decreased cardiac output during ECG monitoring

Neurological	Cardiac	Respiratory	Urinary	Peripheral
• Change in mental status • Light-headedness • Dizziness • Confusion • Loss of consciousness	• Chest pain • Palpitation • Chest discomfort • Enlarged cardiac size • Congestive heart failure	• Difficulty breathing • Shortness of breath • Frothy sputum • Fluid present in lungs • Lung congestion	• Decreased urinary output of less than 30 cc in one hour	• Hypotension • Pale skin • Skin cool and clammy to the touch

How the Patient Is Affected and What You Should Know

Sinus rhythm is the desired rhythm. Patients with this rhythm should have normal cardiac output. Normal cardiac output means that the heart is beating adequately, pumping blood to the body's organs to maintain normal function. Signs and symptoms of adequate cardiac output include an alert and oriented patient with no difficulty breathing, no chest pain or pressure, and a stable blood pressure.

Because this is a normal rhythm, no intervention is necessary. If the patient's rhythm returns to sinus rhythm from another dysrhythmia, it is always important to make sure that the patient is not experiencing problems with low cardiac output, which indicates that the heart is not pumping adequately (see Table 5-2). Any time a patient displays symptoms of low cardiac output, a licensed practitioner needs to be informed for further assessment.

Troubleshooting

Report the Patient Condition, Not the Tracing

The patient you are monitoring is very pale and appears to be breathing very fast. His monitor indicates a sinus rhythm. What should you do?

_____

_____

HIPAA, Law & Ethics

Documenting the ECG Rhythm and Tracing

The ECG rhythm, which is considered a legal document, needs to be included in the patient's medical record. The patient's name, date, and time plus the initials of the person performing the ECG must be identified on each rhythm strip. Documentation of the ECG rhythm and the patient's response help support the reason for the medical treatment.

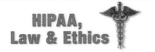 Sinus Bradycardia

Sinus bradycardia is a rhythm of less than 60 beats per minute (see Figure 5-8). Sinus bradycardia originates from the SA node and travels the normal

Figure 5-8 Sinus bradycardia.

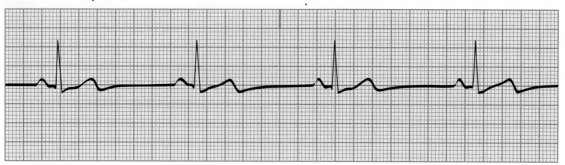

conduction pathway. The only difference between this rhythm and sinus rhythm is that the rate is less than the normal inherent rate of the SA node.

Criteria for Classification

- *Rhythm:* The R-R interval and P-P interval will occur on a regular and constant basis.
- *Rate:* The atrial and ventricular rates will be equal and less than 60 beats per minute.
- *P wave configuration:* The shapes of each of the P waves are identical. There is a P wave in front of each of the QRS complexes. No additional P waves or QRS complexes are noted.
- *PR interval:* The PR interval measurement will be between 0.12 and 0.20 second, which is within normal limits. Each PR interval will be the same.
- *QRS duration and configuration:* The QRS duration and configuration measurement will be between 0.06 and 0.10 second, which is within normal limits. Each QRS duration and configuration will be the same, without any variations from QRS complex to complex.

What's Unique about Sinus Bradycardia?

For sinus bradycardia, the heart rate is less than 60 and all other measurements are within normal limits.

How the Patient Is Affected and What You Should Know

The patient who exhibits sinus bradycardia may or may not experience signs and symptoms of low cardiac output. When administering an ECG to a patient with a slow heart rate, it is important to observe for the symptoms of low cardiac output (see Table 5-2). Remember, though the patient may look all right, he or she can quickly experience difficulties with low cardiac output. When you observe symptoms of low cardiac output, report any findings to a licensed practitioner immediately. This rhythm may require drug administration or application of a pacemaker.

Sinus Tachycardia

Sinus tachycardia is a condition in which the sinoatrial node fires and the electrical impulse travels through the normal conduction pathway but the rate of impulse firing is faster than 100 beats per minute (see Figure 5-9).

Figure 5-9 Sinus tachycardia.

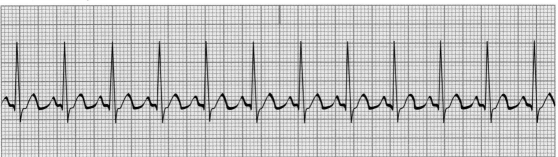

Criteria for Classification

- **Rhythm:** The R-R interval and P-P interval will be equal and constant.
- **Rate:** Both the atrial and ventricular rates will be the same, between 100 and 150 beats per minute.
- **P wave configuration:** The P waves will have the same shape and usually are upright in deflection on the rhythm strip. There will be a P wave in front of every QRS complex.
- **PR interval:** The PR interval measurement will be between 0.12 and 0.20 second. This is within normal limits. Each PR interval will be the same, without any variations.
- **QRS duration and configuration:** The QRS duration and configuration measurement will be between 0.06 and 0.10 second, which is within normal limits. Each QRS duration and configuration will be the same, without any variations from QRS complex to complex.

What's Unique about Sinus Tachycardia?

For sinus tachycardia, the heart rate is greater than 100 and all other measurements are within normal limits.

How the Patient Is Affected and What You Should Know

The effect of this rhythm on the patient depends on the rate of tachycardia above the patient's normal resting heart rate. For example, if the patient's normal resting heart rate is 90 and now the patient is exhibiting a rate of 108 beats per minute after walking the hallway, the tachycardia would be expected and is viewed as the patient's normal response to exercise. However, if the patient's normal heart rate is 60 and it is now 140, the patient is probably experiencing symptoms of low cardiac output. Often the patient will complain of **palpitations** or "heart fluttering" with faster rates. If the patient has had a recent myocardial infarction, sinus tachycardia is considered to be more serious or even life threatening.

When caring for a patient who is experiencing sinus tachycardia, first observe for signs and symptoms of low cardiac output. If evidence of low cardiac output is observed, a licensed practitioner should be notified immediately. Medication may need to be administered by a licensed practitioner.

Figure 5-10 Sinus dyrrhythmia.

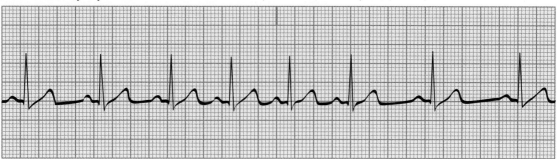

Sinus Dysrhythmia

Sinus dysrhythmia is a condition in which the heart rate remains within normal limits but is influenced by the respiratory cycle and variations of **vagal tone** (a condition in which impulses over the vagus nerve cause a decrease in heart rate), causing the rhythm to be irregular. For instance, when a patient inhales air, the pressure inside the chest cavity increases, causing pressure on the heart, specifically the sinoatrial node. The heart rate will slow with this increase in pressure. As the patient exhales, the chest cavity pressure decreases, allowing the SA node to fire more easily. Therefore, the heart rate will increase during exhalation (see Figure 5-10).

Criteria for Classification

- *Rhythm:* The interval between the P-P and R-R waves will occur at irregular periods.
- *Rate:* Both the atrial and ventricular rates will be the same, between 60 and 100 beats per minute.
- *P wave configuration:* The P waves will have the same shape and usually are upright in deflection on the rhythm strip. There will be a P wave in front of every QRS complex.
- *PR interval:* The PR interval measurement will be between 0.12 and 0.20 second. Each PR interval will be the same, without any variations.
- *QRS duration and configuration:* The QRS duration and configuration measurement will be between 0.06 and 0.10 second. Each QRS duration and configuration will be the same, without any variations from QRS complex to complex.

What's Unique about Sinus Dysrhymia?

For sinus dysrhythmia, the P-P and R-R intervals will progressively widen then narrow following the patient's breathing pattern.

How the Patient Is Affected and What You Should Know

Patients usually show no clinical signs or symptoms with sinus dysrhythmia. If the irregularity is severe enough to decrease the heart rate to the 40s, the patient may complain of palpitations or dizziness. This depends on how slow the heart beats when the SA node is suppressed from the respiratory

Figure 5-11 Sinus arrest.

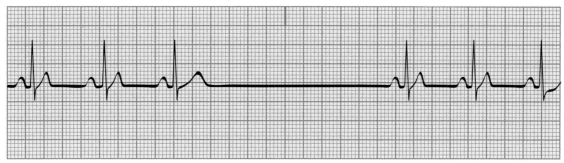

or vagal influences. You should notify the physician or other licensed practitioner when the heart rate slows below 50 or the patient complains of dizziness or palpitations. A copy of the rhythm strip should be mounted on the patient's medical record for documentation.

Sinus Arrest

Sinus arrest occurs when the SA node stops firing, causing a pause in electrical activity. During the pause, no electrical impulse is initiated or sent through the normal conduction system to cause either an atrial or a ventricular contraction (see Figure 5-11).

Criteria for Classification

- *Rhythm:* The interval between the P-P and R-R waves will occur at irregular periods.
- *Rate:* Both the atrial and ventricular rates will be the same. The rate will vary depending on the amount of electrical activity occurring from the sinoatrial node.
- *P wave configuration:* The P waves will have the same shape and usually are upright in deflection on the rhythm strip. There will be a P wave in front of every QRS complex.
- *PR interval:* The PR interval measurement will be between 0.12 and 0.20 second, which is within normal limits. Each PR interval will be the same, without any variations.
- *QRS duration and configuration:* The QRS duration and configuration measurement will be between 0.06 and 0.10 second, which is within normal limits. Each QRS duration and configuration will be the same, without any variations from QRS complex to complex.
- *Length of pause:* The length of pause needs to be measured to determine how long the heart had no rhythm. To measure, place the calipers on the R-R interval around the pause. Once the time frame is determined, calculate the length of time for the pause by multiplying the number of boxes by 0.04 second. The frequency of pauses is also noted because the more frequent the pauses, the more urgent the situation.

  It should be noted that the arrest period may be terminate by an escaped beat from one of the subsidiary pacemakers when the heart rate is less than 60 beats per minute. In this instance, there would be a junctional or ventricular escape beat then resumption of the usual electrical activity.

What Unique about Sinus Arrest?

During sinus arrest, complete cardiac complexes precede and follow the arrest period. There are no nonconducted QRS complexes and no isolated P waves.

How the Patient Is Affected and What You Should Know

The seriousness of sinus arrest depends on the length of the pause. The patient will experience signs and symptoms of decreased cardiac output if the pause is 2 seconds long and occurs on a frequent basis. The pauses may also cause periods of **ischemia** (when cells are deprived of oxygen), hypotension, dizziness, and **syncope** (loss of consciousness).

The patient may initially appear to be asymptomatic (without symptoms) and then develop signs and symptoms of low cardiac output. Therefore, it is important to observe the patient frequently for signs of low cardiac output. Notify a licensed practitioner of these symptoms and provide information about the frequency and length of pauses. The patient will require immediate treatment.

✓ Checkpoint Questions 5-3

1. What rhythm originating in the sinus node is considered "normal"?

   _____

   _____

2. What two rhythms originating in the sinus node only affect the heart rate and how is it affected?

   _____

   _____

3. What rhythm originating in the sinus node is affected by the breathing pattern?

   _____

   _____

 Answer the preceding questions and complete the "Rhythms Originating from the Sinus Node (Sinus Beat)" activity on the student CD under Chapter 5 before you proceed to the next section.

5.4 Rhythms Originating from the Atria

Atrial dysrhythmia is caused by an ectopic beat in either the right or the left atria. However, the atrial origin is outside the SA node, which interrupts the inherent rate of the SA node. The heart works on the principle that the fastest impulse will control the heart rate. Since the atrial ectopic beat is generating electrical impulses faster than the sinoatrial node, the ectopic beat will override the sinoatrial node impulse and cause the atria and ventricles to depolarize. Dysrhythmias that are caused by the atrial ectopic site include premature atrial complexes, atrial tachycardia, atrial flutter, and atrial fibrillation.

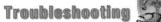

A patient is in sinus arrest that lasts longer than 6 seconds. This indicates that no electrical current is traveling through the cardiac conduction system and is known as **asystole**. What should you do?

_____

_____

Atrial dysrhythmias occur from conditions that cause pressure on the atria such as damage to the atria from myocardial infarction, valvular problems, or **neurological** influences (pertaining to the nervous system). When the area is stressed or damaged, the cells become unstable and the electrical state may cause depolarization to occur more easily.

Premature Atrial Complexes

Premature atrial complexes (PACs) are electrical impulses that originate in the atria and initiate an early impulse that interrupts the inherent regular rhythm (see Figure 5-12).

Criteria for Classification

- *Rhythm:* The regularity between the P-P interval and R-R interval is constant with the exception of the early complexes. There will be a section of the rhythm that is regular and occasionally an early complex.
- *Rate:* The rates of the atria and ventricles will usually be within normal limits of 60 to 100, depending on the frequency of the PACs.
- *P wave configuration:* The P waves will have the same configuration and shape. The early beat will have a different shape than the rest of the P waves on the strip. This P wave may be flattened, notched, **biphasic** (have two phases), or otherwise unusual. It may even be hidden within the T wave of the preceding complex. Evidence that the P wave is hidden within the T wave includes a notch in the T wave, a pointed shape, or being taller than the other T waves.
- *PR interval:* The PR interval will measure within normal limits of 0.12 to 0.20 second. The early beat will probably have a different PR measurement than the normal complexes but will be within normal limits.
- *QRS duration and configuration:* The QRS duration and configuration will be within normal limits of 0.06 to 0.10 second.

Figure 5-12 Premature atrial complex (PAC).

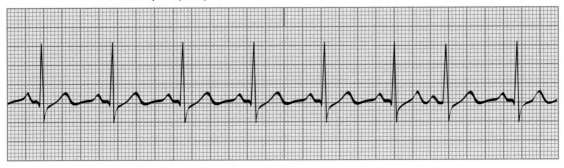

What's Unique about Premature Atrial Complexes?

A premature atrial complex is a beat earlier than it should be with a positively deflected P wave.

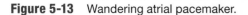

Determine the underlying rhythm of sinus rhythm, sinus bradycardia, sinus tachycardia, or sinus dysrhythmia when identifying PACs. The rhythm strip must be labeled with this underlying rhythm and the type of PAC. An example of this terminology is "sinus rhythm with trigeminal PACs" (**trigeminy** refers to a pattern in which every third complex is a premature beat).

How the Patient Is Affected and What You Should Know

With each PAC, the atria do not achieve the maximum blood capacity prior to contraction. This lack of blood causes a decrease in cardiac output and less volume in the ventricles prior to ventricular contraction. Therefore, in the patient who has prior cardiac disease, frequent PACs can cause the patient to experience symptoms of low cardiac output.

When caring for a patient with PACs, observe the patient for signs and symptoms of low cardiac output. Monitoring the amount or frequency of PACs is essential. The patient may complain of palpitations from the early beats. The severity of the patient's complaints is related to the frequency of the PACs. In addition, frequent PACs may indicate that a more serious atrial dysrhythmia may follow. The more frequent occurrence indicates that the ectopic **focus** (cardiac cell that functions as an ectopic beat) may continue and take control of the heart rate. Any observation of low cardiac output should be communicated to a licensed practitioner for appropriate treatment.

Wandering Atrial Pacemaker

Wandering atrial pacemaker (WAP) is a rhythm in which the pacemaker site shifts between the SA node, atria, and/or the AV junction. The P wave configuration changes in appearance during the pacemaker shift. At least three different P wave configurations in the same lead indicate a wandering atrial pacemaker (see Figure 5-13).

Figure 5-13 Wandering atrial pacemaker.

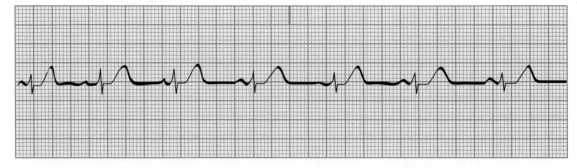

Criteria for Classification

- **Rhythm:** Slightly irregular
- **Rate:** Should be within normal limits of 60 to 100 beats per minute
- **P wave configuration:** Continuous change in appearance
- **PR interval:** Varies
- **QRS duration and configuration:** Usually within normal limits

---

What's Unique about Wandering Atrial Pacemaker Rhythm?

WAP has a changing P wave configuration with at least three variations in one lead. The rhythm may be irregular.

How the Patient Is Affected and What You Should Know

WAP is a normal finding in children, older adults, and well-conditioned athletes and does not usually cause clinical signs and symptoms. However, it may also be related to some types of organic heart disease and drug toxicity.

Multifocal Atrial Tachycardia

Multifocal atrial tachycardia (MAT) has a P wave that changes from beat to beat and a heart rate of 120 to 150 (see Figure 5-14). It has the same characteristics as wandering atrial pacemaker (WAP) and is frequently mistaken for atrial fibrillation. It can be distinguished by looking closely for visible changing P waves.

Criteria for Classification

- **Rhythm:** Irregular
- **Rate:** Between 101 and 150 beats per minute
- **P wave configuration:** P waves change in appearance from beat to beat. They may be upright, rounded, notched, inverted, biphasic, or buried in the QRS complex.
- **PR interval:** Varies
- **QRS duration and configuration:** Normal in duration and all complexes look alike

Figure 5-14 Multifocal atrial tachycardia.

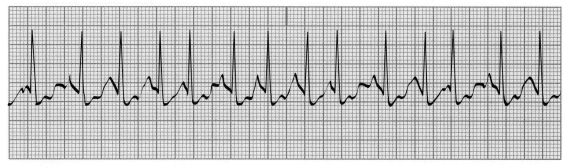

How the Patient Is Affected and What You Should Know

MAT is usually triggered by an acute attack of emphysema, congestive heart failure (CHF), or acute mitral valve regurgitation. This rhythm should be reported to the licensed practitioner, and the patient's vital signs and condition should be monitored.

Atrial Flutter

Atrial flutter (A flutter) occurs when a rapid impulse originates in the atrial tissue. The ectopic focus may be originating from ischemic areas of the heart with enhanced **automaticity** (ability to initiate an electrical current) or from a reentry pathway. A reentry pathway is an extra pathway that has developed where a group of cells will generate an impulse faster than the SA node. This impulse then follows a route that allows the impulse to reach the AV node quicker than the normal conduction pathway. The reentry pathway is similar to finding a shortcut to work or school to bypass the normal traffic route to get you to your destination faster. The electrical current or rhythm is recorded in a characteristic sawtooth pattern (see Figure 5-15). This atrial activity is called flutter (F) waves. Most often this is a transient dysrhythmia that will lead to more serious atrial dysrhythmia if not treated.

Criteria for Classification

- **Rhythm:** The P-P interval or flutter-to-flutter waves will be regular. The interval set with the calipers will stay constant throughout the rhythm. The R-R interval is usually irregular, but occasionally it may be regular in pattern. The regularity of the R-R interval will depend on the ability of the AV node to limit impulses to ventricles.
- **Rate:** The atrial rate will be between 250 and 350 beats per minute.
- **P wave configuration:** P waves are not seen, and only flutter waves are present. These flutter waves resemble a "sawtooth" or "picket fence." They will be seen best in leads II, III, and aVF. The correlation between

Figure 5-15 Atrial flutter.

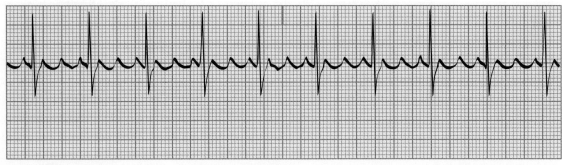

P waves and QRS complexes no longer exists. There will be more flutter waves than QRS complexes, and presence of "F" or flutter waves.

- *PR interval:* No identifiable P wave exists, so the PR interval cannot be measured.
- *QRS duration and configuration:* The QRS duration will be within normal limits of 0.06 to 0.10 second.

What's Unique about Atrial Flutter?

Atrial flutter has a "sawtooth" atrial pattern between the QRS complexes.

How the Patient Is Affected and What You Should Know

The **atrial kick,** which occurs when blood is ejected into the ventricles by the atria immediately prior to ventricular systole, is no longer present since the atria do not contract completely, followed by a delay in the ventricular contraction. This loss in atrial kick contributes to a 10% to 30% decrease in cardiac output. Some patients may tolerate this if the heart rate is within normal limits of 60 to 100 beats per minute. But once the heart rate increases significantly and loss of the atrial kick occurs, the patient will demonstrate signs and symptoms of low cardiac output.

When atrial flutter occurs, notify the licensed practitioner to implement a treatment plan, which usually includes oxygen therapy to ensure adequate supply to the vital organs. The patient is monitored continuously to determine if the rhythm converts to a sinus rhythm or progresses to atrial fibrillation. A continuous rhythm strip is needed to document if any changes occurred as a result of the medical intervention. Always indicate on the rhythm strip the type of intervention that is being implemented. The ECG strips are then mounted and saved in the patient's medical record or chart.

Atrial Fibrillation

Atrial fibrillation (A fib.) occurs when electrical impulses come from areas of reentry pathways or multiple ectopic foci. Each electrical impulse results in depolarization of only a small group of atrial cells rather than the whole atria. This results in the atria not contracting as a whole, causing it to quiver, similar to a bowl of Jell-O™ when shaken. Multiple atrial activity is recorded as a chaotic wave, often with the appearance of fine scribbles (see Figure 5-16). No P wave can be identified. The waveform of the chaotic "scribbles" is referred to as fibrillatory waves or "f" waves.

Criteria for Classification

- *Rhythm:* The P-P interval is unable to be determined because of the fibrillatory waves or f waves. The R-R interval is irregular.
- *Rate:* Atrial rate, if measurable, will be from 375 to 700 beats per minute. It is difficult to determine the atrial rates because each fibrillatory wave is not easy to identify or measure. The ventricular rate is initially

Figure 5-16   Atrial fibrillation.

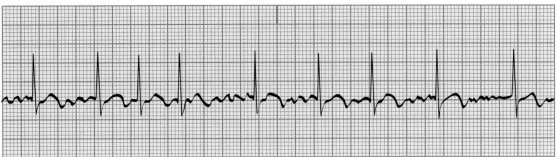

between 160 and 180 beats per minute prior to administering medication. Once medication is provided, the ventricular rate is considered under control if the rate is between 60 and 100 beats per minute.

- *P wave configuration:* The P waves cannot be identified. There is chaotic electrical activity, or "f" waves may be seen.
- *PR interval:* The PR interval cannot be measured, since the P wave is not identifiable.
- *QRS duration and configuration:* The QRS duration and configuration will be within normal limits of 0.06 to 0.10 second and irregular.

What's Unique about Atrial Fibrillation?

Atrial fibrillation shows chaotic disorganized activity between QRS complexes.

How the Patient Is Affected and What You Should Know

The patient will exhibit signs and symptoms of decreased cardiac output. The patient usually has limited cardiac function because of preexisting cardiac conditions, so with the loss of atrial kick, the patient's cardiac output will decrease significantly. Once the heart rate is controlled within the range of 60 to 100 beats per minute, the patient may be able to tolerate the loss of the atrial kick.

Blood will begin to collect in the atria because they are not contracting completely, allowing the opportunity for a clot or thrombus to form. Therefore, the patient has an increased risk of developing and sending an embolism (traveling blood clot) out into the body's systemic circulation, which can then migrate to other vital organs, such as the lungs or brain. The patient may develop a cerebral vascular accident (CVA), myocardial infarction (MI), pulmonary embolism, renal infarction, or an embolism in any place that the arterial blood is transported. Essentially, the heart is playing Russian roulette with us because there is no way to predict where the embolism will travel in the body to cause serious damage or even sudden death.

Patients who exhibit atrial fibrillation must be observed for low cardiac output. The rhythm needs to be monitored closely as the medication or electrical cardioversion is attempted. Report any complications or vital sign changes to the licensed practitioner immediately.

1. The patient has coronary artery disease. How would you expect PACs to affect this patient?

   _____

   _____

2. What treatment is usually indicated for patients with atrial flutter?

   _____

   _____

3. What is the best way to describe the rhythm pattern for atrial fibrillation?

   _____

   _____

4. Which rhythm is considered more serious, MAT or WAP, and why?

   _____

   _____

 Answer the preceding questions and complete the "Rhythms Originating from the Atria" activity on the student CD under Chapter 5 before you proceed to the next section.

5.5 Rhythms Originating from the Atrial-Junction Node

The atrioventricular node is sometimes referred to as the AV junction or AV tissue. Though abnormal, these AV node cells, which possess the property of automaticity, can function as a pacemaker. The inherent rate of the AV node is between 40 and 60 beats per minute. When the AV node instead of the SA node initiates the electrical impulse, the rhythm is referred to as a junctional dysrhythmia. With junctional rhythms, it is important to understand that the electrical current is initiated from the AV junction. Junctional rhythms are suggestive of more serious conditions with the electrical conduction system in the heart. The AV node is the backup pacemaker for the heart after the SA node. Junctional rhythm, accelerated junctional rhythm, and junctional tachycardia are all conditions in which the SA node has been injured and the AV node functions as the pacemaker of the heart.

Premature Junctional Complex

A premature junctional complex (PJC) is a single early electrical impulse that originates in the atrioventricular junction. It occurs before the next expected sinus impulse, causing an irregularity in the rhythm (see Figure 5-17).

Criteria for Classification

- **Rhythm:** May be occasionally irregular or frequently irregular depending upon the number of PJCs present
- **Rate:** Will depend upon the underlying rhythm

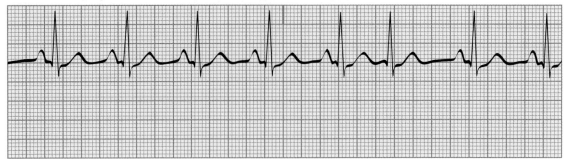

- *P wave configuration:* The P wave is inverted and may immediately precede or follow the QRS complex.
- *PR interval:* Will be shorter than normal if the P wave precedes the QRS complex, absent if the P wave is buried in the QRS.
- *QRS duration and configuration:* The QRS duration and configuration will be between 0.06 and 0.10 second, which is within normal limits.

What's Unique about Premature Junctional Complex?

PJCs have an irregular rhythm and the P wave is inverted and may appear before, during, or after the QRS complex.

How the Patient Is Affected and What You Should Know

When the patient has a healthy heart, isolated PJCs cause no signs or symptoms. If PJCs occur more than four to six per minute, this warns of a more serious condition. An irregular pulse would be noted, and the patient may experience hypotension due to low cardiac output.

Junctional Rhythm

Junctional rhythm also known as junctional escape rhythm originates at atrioventricular junctional tissue, producing retrograde (backward) depolarization of atrial tissue, and, at the same time, stimulates the depolarization of ventricles (see Figure 5-18).

Figure 5-18 Junctional rhythm.

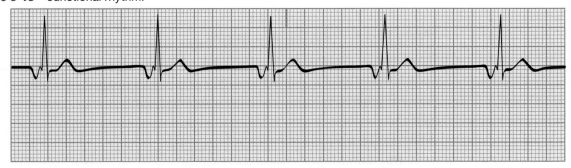

Criteria for Classification

- **Rhythm:** The P-P and R-R intervals are regular and at similar intervals. The P-P interval may be difficult to measure due to the location of the P wave.
- **Rate:** If the P wave is identifiable, the rate will be 40 to 60 beats per minute. The ventricular rate will be 40 to 60 beats per minute.
- **P wave configuration:** The P wave is usually inverted and may precede, follow, or fall within the QRS complex. It may not be visible at all on the rhythm strip.
- **PR interval:** If the P wave is before the QRS complex, the PR interval will measure less than 0.12 second and will be constant. If the P wave is not before the QRS complex, the PR interval cannot be determined. This is because this P wave is not associated with the next QRS complex.
- **QRS duration and configuration:** The QRS duration and configuration will be within normal limits of 0.06 to 0.10 second.

What's Unique about Junctional Rhythm?

A junctional rhythm may have an inverted or absent P wave or a P wave that follows the QRS complex.

How the Patient Is Affected and What You Should Know

The patient has a slower heart rate than normal and loses the atrial kick due to the shortening of the interval between the atrial depolarization and ventricular depolarization. These conditions cause the patient to exhibit symptoms of low cardiac output. Common signs and symptoms of low cardiac output displayed include **hypotension** (low blood pressure) and altered mental status such as confusion or disorientation. Observe for symptoms and monitor the ECG tracing in case a more serious dysrhythmia occurs. Report the presence of junctional rhythm and your observations of the patient to a licensed practitioner for appropriate medical treatment.

Checkpoint Question 5-5

1. What are differences between a PJC rhythm and a junctional rhythm?

_____

_____

 Answer the preceding question and complete the "Rhythms Originating from the Atrial-Junction Node" activity on the student CD under Chapter 5 before you proceed to the next section.

Figure 5-19 Supraventricular tachycardia.

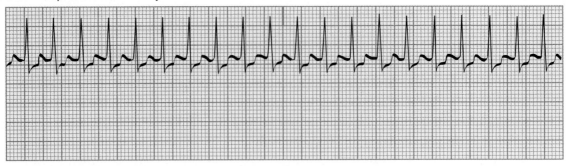

5.6 Supraventricular Dysrhythmias

A supraventricular tachycardia (SVT) is a classification of rapid heartbeats, usually occurring at a rate greater than 150 beats per minute (see Figure 5-19). **Supraventricular** refers to an ectopic focus originating above the ventricles, in the atria, or junctional region of the heart. The heart is beating so fast that it is difficult to determine if the source of origin is from the sinus node, atria, or the AV junction. Because the heart rate is so rapid, the atria are contracting as soon as the ventricles are relaxing. This causes the P waves (atrial contraction) to become difficult to identify, because they may occur at the same time as the T waves (ventricle relaxation). Rhythms that fall into this category are identified in Table 5-3.

The primary difficulty in classifying the actual rhythm is identifying where the tachycardia originates. The P wave may appear before, after, or during the QRS complex, depending on the origin. The PR interval measurement is difficult to assess because you cannot often see the initial upswing of the P wave. Frequently, the licensed practitioner will request the paper speed be increased to pull the cardiac complexes apart for further analysis. However, be sure to mark the tracing if this is done.

Criteria for Classification

- **Rhythm:** The ventricular (R-R) rhythm is usually regular or with minimal irregularity from R-R interval. The atrial rhythm may or may not be seen. This is because other electrical activity is occurring at the same time. Remember, the ECG will record only the activity it "sees" in each lead. The atrial activity is small compared to ventricular activity; therefore, the ventricular activity is the largest amount of energy seen when the ECG tracing is recorded. Depending on whether the P waves are seen, you may not be able to determine regular P waves. If identifiable, they are usually regular.

TABLE 5-3 Dysrhythmias Associated with Supraventricular Tachycardia

Sinus Node	Atrium	Junctional
Sinus tachycardia	Atrial flutter	Junctional tachycardia
	Atrial fibrillation	

- **Rate:** The ventricular rate is 150 to 350 beats per minute. The atrial rate will be difficult to determine when P waves are unidentifiable.
- **P wave configuration:** The P waves are usually not identified when the heart rate is this rapid. Remember that when the heart rate increases, the time interval between atrial contraction and ventricular relaxation decreases. Therefore, if there is a P wave present, it may occur simultaneously with the T wave and may be buried within it. The P wave may occur before, during, or after the QRS complex.
- **PR interval:** Usually the PR interval is unable to be determined because the beginning of the P wave cannot be clearly identified.
- **QRS duration and configuration:** The QRS measurement is considered within normal limits when measured at 0.06 to 0.10 second.

What's Unique about Supraventricular dysrhythmias?

Supraventricular dysrhythmias are rate dependent with a rate of greater than 150 beats per minute.

How the Patient Is Affected and What You Should Know

There are various supraventricular dysrhythmias, all of which may cause the patient to exhibit the same signs and symptoms. The patient may be in either a stable or an unstable condition. The stable patient (one without signs and symptoms of decreased cardiac output) may only complain of palpitations and state, "I'm just not feeling right" or "My heart is fluttering." When the patient's condition is *unstable,* he or she may experience any symptom of low cardiac output, which is reflective of the heart not pumping effectively to other body systems. Many patients may present initially with a stable condition and then a few minutes later experience unstable symptoms such as those presented in Table 5-2.

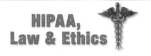

HIPAA, Law & Ethics

Scope of Practice

Your role regarding evaluation of the rhythm strip and assessment of the patient will depend on your training and place of employment. Working outside of your scope of practice is illegal, and you could be held liable for performing tasks that are not part of your role as a health care professional.

Observe the patient for signs and symptoms of low cardiac output. Signs, symptoms, and rhythm changes need to be communicated quickly to a licensed practitioner for appropriate medical treatment. Because tachycardia severely deprives the heart of oxygen, treatment should begin as early as possible. It is difficult to predict how long a patient's heart can beat at a rapid rate before it begins to affect the other body systems.

1. What are the rate and the origination point of a supraventricular tachycardia?

   _____

   _____

2. What might you be asked to do when a patient has a supraventricular dysrhythmia?

   _____

   _____

3. Name the dysrhythmias associated with supraventricular tachycardia.

   _____

   _____

Answer the preceding questions and complete the "Supraventricular Dysrhythmias" activity on the student CD under Chapter 5 before you proceed to the next section.

5.7 Heart Block Rhythms

In heart block rhythms, the electrical current has difficulty traveling along the normal conduction pathway, causing a delay in or absence of ventricular depolarization. The degree of blockage is dependent on the area affected and the cause of the delay or blockage. There are three levels of heart blocks. The P-P interval is regular with all heart blocks.

First Degree Atrioventricular Block

First degree AV block is a *delay* in electrical conduction from the SA node to the AV node, usually around the AV node, which prevents an electrical impulse from traveling to the ventricular conduction system (see Figure 5-20). The condition is similar to being in a traffic jam. You still arrive at your destination, but it takes you longer to get there. Electrical current from the SA node will still stimulate ventricular depolarization, but the time it takes to arrive in the ventricles is longer than normal.

Figure 5-20   First degree AV block.

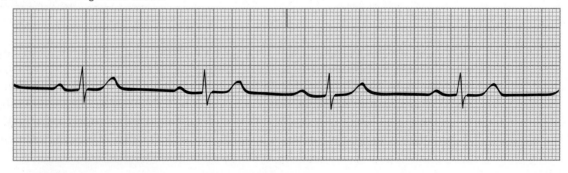

Criteria for Classification

- **Rhythm:** The regularity between the P-P interval and the R-R interval is constant.
- **Rate:** The rate of the atria and ventricles will usually be within normal limits of 60 to 100 beats per minute.
- **P wave configuration:** The P waves will have the same configuration and shape. Each QRS complex will have a P wave before it. There will be the same number of P waves as QRS complexes.
- **PR interval:** The PR interval will be greater than 0.20 second.
- **QRS duration and configuration:** The QRS duration and configuration will be within normal limits of 0.06 to 0.10 second.

What's Unique about First Degree AV Block?

With first degree atrioventricular block, the PR interval is constant and measures greater than 0.20 second.

How the Patient Is Affected and What You Should Know

The patient will be able to maintain normal cardiac output. No change in the patient should occur with this rhythm. Monitor and observe for further degeneration and development of other heart blocks and report if they occur. It is important to observe the **cardiac output parameters**—to assess the blood supply to the vital organs—and to determine how well the patient is tolerating the dysrhythmia.

Second Degree Atrioventricular (AV) Block, Mobitz I (Wenckebach)

Second degree heart block has some **blocked or nonconducted** electrical **impulses** from the SA node to the ventricles at the atrioventricular junction region. The impulses from the atrium are regular but the conduction through the AV node gets delayed where the impulse does not get to the ventricles, therefore being blocked. However, some electrical impulses are still being conducted along the normal conduction pathway. Second degree heart blocks are the only blocks with an irregular ventricular response.

There are currently two different types of second degree heart blocks, which were first discovered by Dr. Mobitz. Dr. Wenckebach further investigated the rhythm and was able to identify a similar blockage pattern, but it was different from the one Dr. Mobitz observed. The rhythm Dr. Wenckebach observed was specifically labeled second degree atrioventricular block, Mobitz I, although it is often referred to as a Wenckebach rhythm. It is caused when diseased or injured atrioventricular node tissue conducts the electrical impulse to the ventricular conduction pathway with increasing difficulty, causing a delay in time until one of the atrial impulses fails to be conducted or is blocked. After the dropped atrial impulse, the atrioventricular node resets itself to be able to handle future impulses more quickly and then progressively gets more difficult until it drops or is blocked again. This pattern will repeat itself (see Figure 5-21).

Figure 5-21 Second degree AV block, Mobitz I. (Wenckebach)

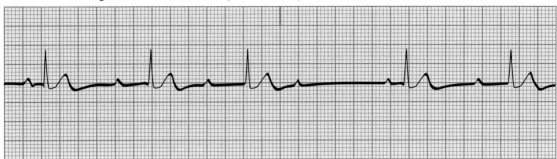

Criteria for Classification

- **Rhythm:** The P-P interval will be regular. The R-R interval will be irregular due to the blocked impulse(s).
- **Rate:** Atrial rate will be within normal limits. The ventricular rate will be slower than the atrial rate.
- **P wave configuration:** The P wave configuration will be normal size with an upright P wave. There will be a P wave for every QRS complex, but there will be extra P waves.
- **PR interval:** The PR interval will vary from one measurement to the next. The PR interval will be progressively longer with each subsequent conducted P wave until the QRS wave is dropped. The PR interval will be short, and then the cycle will begin again.
- **QRS duration and configuration:** The QRS duration and configuration should be within normal limits of 0.06 to 0.10 second.

What's Unique about Second Degree AV Block Mobitz I (Wenckebach)?

A Mobitz I rhythm has a cyclical extending PR interval until the QRS is dropped. Then the cycle begins again (irregular ventricular response).

How the Patient Is Affected and What You Should Know

The patient may or may not exhibit symptoms of decreased cardiac output, depending on the heart rate of the ventricles. As this rate decreases and reaches levels of 40 beats per minute or lower, the patient will show signs and symptoms of low cardiac output. This rhythm is usually due to inflammation around the atrioventricular node, and it is often a temporary condition that will resolve itself and return to a normal heart rhythm.

Since treatment is based on how the patient is tolerating the rhythm, the patient is observed for signs and symptoms of low cardiac output. If the patient is experiencing difficulties, a licensed practitioner administers medication; if not, the patient is monitored for further progression to third degree heart block.

Figure 5-22 Mobitz second degree type II.

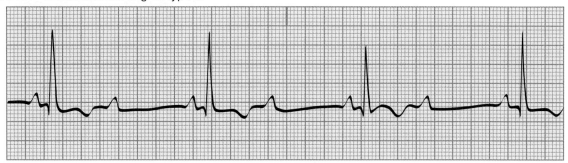

Second Degree Atrioventricular (AV) Block, Mobitz Type II

Second degree atrioventricular block, Mobitz II, is often referred to as the classical heart block because it was the first rhythm observed to have an occasional dropped complex (see Figure 5-22). The atrioventricular node selects which electrical impulses it will block. No pattern or reason for the dropping of the QRS complex exists. Frequently this dysrhythmia will progress to third degree atrioventricular block.

Criteria for Classification

- **Rhythm:** The P-P interval will be regular. The R-R interval will be irregular due to the blocked impulse(s).
- **Rate:** Atrial rate will be within normal limits. The ventricular rate will be slower than the atrial rate. The atrial and ventricular rates will not be the same.
- **P wave configuration:** The P wave configuration will be normal, with a normal size and upright wave. There will be a P wave for every QRS complex, but there will be more P waves than QRS complexes.
- **PR interval:** The PR interval is constant and will remain constant even after the QRS drop occurs.
- **QRS duration and configuration:** The QRS duration and configuration should be within normal limits of 0.06 to 0.10 second.

What's Unique about Second Degree (AV) Block, Mobitz Type II?

A Mobitz II rhythm has a constant PR interval with blocked QRS complexes (irregular ventricular response).

How the Patient Is Affected and What You Should Know

Observe the patient for signs and symptoms of low cardiac output since this rhythm frequently will progress very quickly to a third degree atrioventricular block or complete heart block (CHB), usually within seconds. Recognition of the classical block pattern versus the Wenckebach pattern is essential. See Table 5-4 for differences between second degree heart blocks. The classical block is more critical and can quickly lead to a complete heart block and a Code Blue situation. When your patient is experiencing second degree heart block, Mobitz II, you should immediately report it to a licensed

TABLE 5-4 Differences Between Second Degree Heart Blocks

Type of Heart Block	PR Interval	Etiology	Treatment
Second degree AV block, Mobitz I (Wenckebach)	Varies from one complex to another; will reset itself after the dropped complex	Temporary	May resolve itself; observe cardiac output and wait until the PR intervals vary and the dropped QRS complexes occur
Second degree AV block, Mobitz II (classical block)	Constant PR interval throughout the rhythm strip	Chronic situation	Quickly leads to a complete heart block, a life-threatening situation that needs immediate attention: call 911 or Code Blue

practitioner; and, if trained, you should prepare for a Code Blue and application of a temporary external pacemaker.

Troubleshooting **Mobitz I versus Mobitz II**

To quickly determine the difference between a second degree, Mobitz I (Wenckebach), and a second degree, Mobitz II (classical rhythm), atrioventricular block, look for the dropped beat indicated by a missing QRS complex. For the Wenckebach rhythm, the PR interval in front of the dropped QRS complex will be longer than the PR interval after the dropped QRS complex. Remember the mnemonic "Lengthen, Lengthen, drop equals Wenckebach." For the classical rhythm, the PR interval in front and behind the dropped QRS complex will be constant. Both rhythms should be reported; however, the classical rhythm is a critical condition, unlike the Wenckebach rhythm, which will usually resolve itself.

What does the mnemonic "Lengthen, Lengthen, drop equals Wenckebach" mean?

_____

_____

Third Degree Atrioventricular (AV) Block

Third degree atrioventricular block is also known as *third degree heart block* or *complete heart block* (CHB). All electrical impulses originating above the ventricles are blocked and prevented from reaching the ventricles. There is no correlation between atrial and ventricular depolarization. As a result, there will be noticeable and suspicious disassociation properties; namely the P-P and R-R intervals. Although the intervals are regular when measured, the atria and ventricles will be firing at completely different rates. This is due to the "block," and as a result the ventricular rate will be slower than the atrial rate (see Figure 5-23).

The rate of the ventricular response and the configuration of the QRS complex will be dependent upon the level of the block. If the block is low in the bundle of His, the pacemaker would come from the slow (20 to 40 beats

Figure 5-23 Third degree AV block. (Complete Heart Block)

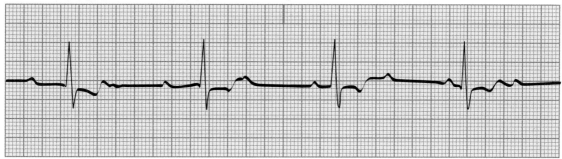

per minute) Purkinje network. The QRS complex in this instance would measure 0.12 second or greater.

If the block is higher and the impulse causing ventricular depolarization is coming from the area of the AV tissue, then the rate is likely to be 40 to 60 beats per minute and the QRS complex will present with a "normal to narrow" appearance measuring 0.06 to 0.10 second. The ventricular rate and QRS configurations are keys indicating the level of the heart block.

Criteria for Classification

- *Rhythm:* The P-P inteval is regular. The R-R interval is also regular, but the P-P and R-R intervals will be different.
- *Rate:* The atrial rate will be within normal limits of 60 to 100 beats per minute. The ventricular rate is slow, between 20 and 40 beats per minute.
- *P wave configuration:* P waves will be of normal size and configuration, but the location may be buried within the QRS, either before or after the QRS complex. There will be no correlation seen between the P waves and the QRS complex. More P waves will be noted than QRS complexes, and not every P wave will have a QRS complex following it.
- *PR interval:* Appearance of a pattern consisting of a long PR interval followed by a short PR interval is a clue that a complete heart block exists.
- *QRS duration and configuration:* The QRS duration and configuration will be the same but the measurements may be either within normal limits or wide, depending on the area of the blockage.

What's Unique about Third Degree (Complete) Heart Block?

In third degree atrioventricular block, the P-P and R-R intervals are regular (constant) but firing at different rates.

How the Patient Is Affected and What You Should Know

The patient has lost coordination between the atria and ventricles; therefore, the atrial kick is lost. Along with the loss of atrial kick and reduced heart rate, the patient will exhibit signs and symptoms of low cardiac output. Often the patient will be unconscious and require immediate medical intervention.

In a situation where the patient is in third degree AV block, your first responsibility is to observe the patient for symptoms of low cardiac output. If the patient displays any signs and symptoms, a licensed practitioner needs to be contacted immediately. Initiating a Code Blue procedure makes this contact. A temporary pacemaker should be available and ready for application as deemed necessary by the licensed practitioner. All rhythm strips should be mounted and identified in the patient's medical record as documentation of the dysrhythmia.

Checkpoint Questions 5-7

1. Name the heart block rhythms described in this section. Which one is most serious?

   _____

   _____

2. How can you tell the difference between a Mobitz I and Mobitz II heart block?

   _____

   _____

3. What should you do if the patient has a third degree heart block?

   _____

   _____

 Answer the preceding questions and complete the "Heart Block Rhythms" activity on the student CD under Chapter 5 before you proceed to the next section.

5.8 Bundle Branch Block Dysrhythmias

Bundle branch blocks occur when one or both of the ventricular pathways are damaged or delayed due to cardiac disease, drugs, or other conditions. When an area of one of the bundle branches is damaged, electrical current will not be able to travel through that tissue to reach the myocardial tissue in its usual fashion. Current will travel down the good bundle and will activate the myocardial tissue in that corresponding ventricle only. The other ventricle must then receive the impulse as current travels from one cell to the next until the entire myocardial contraction occurs. It is similar to the knocking down of a line of dominoes where each domino represents a cardiac cell. The cell will not contract until the next cell delivers the energy.

Current not traveling the normal pathways will take longer to achieve the full ventricular contraction. This longer time frame is similar to driving a car to a specific destination and having to find an alternate route or detour when the road is closed. This is what happens to the current traveling through the heart's conduction pathway when it has a blocked bundle branch. The increased length of time is reflected in the QRS duration. Remember that the QRS duration is a measurement of just how long it takes for current to travel through ventricular myocardial tissue.

When a patient has a right bundle branch block (RBBB), the impulse will travel down the conduction pathway normally until after the bundle of His.

Figure 5-24 Ventricular conduction with a right bundle branch block.

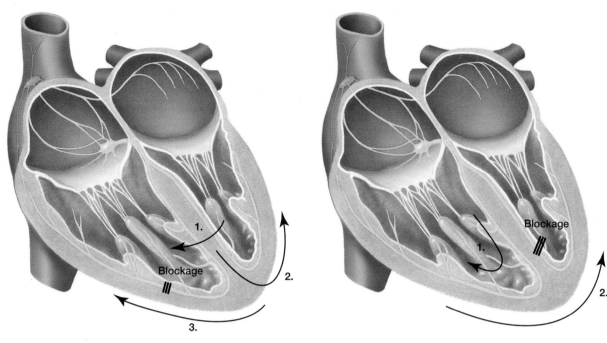

A. Ventricular conduction with an RBBB
1. The septum is depolarized normally.
2. The left ventricle is activated.
3. The current travels to the right ventricle until there is complete ventricular contraction.

B. Ventricular conduction with an LBBB
1. Current travels down the right bundle branch to cause right vntricle contraction.
2. The current moves to the left ventricle causing the septum to be activated abnormally in a right-to-left fashion.

Since the right side of the conduction pathway is blocked, current must travel down the left bundle branch to activate the ventricles (see Figure 5-24A).

The left bundle branch block (LBBB) will have the left conduction pathway blocked. Current travels down the right bundle branch to cause the right ventricle, the septum, then the left ventricle to contract (see Figure 5-24B).

The bundle branch block classification provides additional information about another dysrhythmia. Information regarding a bundle branch block is extra data included with the basic rhythm classification. Typically the basic rhythm will be a rhythm that originates from above the ventricles. The rhythm has all the basic properties of sinus rhythms or atrial dysrhythmias with the exception of a wide QRS complex. The discovery of a wide QRS complex is the clue to further investigate for the bundle branch block. For example, the patient may be experiencing sinus rhythm with a left bundle branch block (SR with LBBB). The basic rhythm must always be determined with the distinction of a right bundle branch block or left bundle branch block present.

Criteria for Classification

Characteristics of the right and left bundle branch block will be similar over monitoring leads I, II, and III. Specific characteristics of the right or left bundle branch will be present when monitoring with leads V1 to V6. Although bundle branch block (BBB) is seen in the precordial leads, to distinguish RBBB from LBBB, lead VI is referenced. If the QRS is positively deflected, it is an RBBB. If the QRS is negative, it is an LBBB.

- **Rhythm:** The regularity or irregularity will depend on the underlying rhythm. Sinus or atrial is usually the underlying rhythm, with both regular and irregular rhythm patterns possible.
- **Rate:** The atrial and ventricular rates will depend on the basic rhythm.
- **P wave configuration:** The shape, configuration, deflection, and coordination with the QRS complex will depend on the basic rhythm.
- **PR interval:** The PR interval will be a normal measurement of 0.12 to 0.20 second.
- **QRS duration and configuration:** The QRS measurement will be 0.12 second or greater in length. The widening of the QRS duration indicates the presence of a bundle branch block.

How the Patient Is Affected and What You Should Know

The patient will exhibit the normal effects of the basic rhythm he or she is experiencing. For example, if the rhythm is sinus tachycardia, the patient will exhibit the sign and symptoms of a fast heart rate. A bundle branch block condition can further deteriorate to the development of another bundle branch block. If the current becomes totally blocked and current cannot reach the myocardium, this is considered a complete heart block.

Initially, you will observe a widening of the QRS complex, which indicates the presence of a bundle branch block. This should be reported to a licensed practitioner immediately. The patient will need to be monitored further by the licensed practitioner to determine whether an RBBB or LBBB pattern is present, and the patient's condition should be observed for deterioration. All patients must have a 12-lead ECG to document the bundle branch block. If further degeneration of the conduction system occurs, treatment may be a pacemaker. Pacemakers are applied to the external skin for a temporary condition for only 24 hours at a time. The patient may end up in a Code Blue situation and/or needing a permanent pacemaker.

Checkpoint Questions 5-8

1. What happens when one or both of the ventricular pathways are not functioning properly due to damage or a delay from cardiac disease, drugs, or other conditions?

   _____

   _____

2. Describe the electrical conduction for the RBBB and an LBBB.

   _____

   _____

   _____

 Answer the preceding questions and complete the "Bundle Branch Block Dysrhythmias" activity on the student CD under Chapter 5 before you proceed to the next section.

Figure 5-25   Premature ventricular complexes

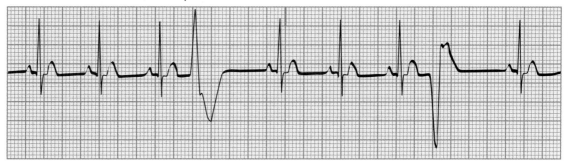

5.9 Rhythms Originating from the Ventricles

As discussed in Chapter 2, the ventricle pacemaker cells are found at the Purkinje fibers (see Figure 2-9). This pacemaker is the last of the group of inherent pacemaker cells within the heart. The rate of automaticity is between 20 and 40 beats per minute. Current is initiated within the Purkinje fibers and spreads the electrical stimulation from one ventricular cell to the next. Since current is not traveling down the normal ventricular conduction pathway to activate both the right and left ventricles simultaneously, it will take longer than normal to depolarize the ventricles. A QRS duration and configuration measurement of 0.12 second or greater suggests that this cell-by-cell stimulation of electrical current is occurring to depolarize the ventricles.

Premature Ventricular Complexes

A premature ventricular complex (PVC) is caused by an ectopic beat that occurs early in the cycle and originates from the ventricles (see Figure 5-25). Table 5-5 shows the various types of premature ventricular complexes.

TABLE 5-5   Types of Premature Ventricular Complexes

Unifocal	Early beat (has similar shape and shape suggesting only one irritable focus present)
Multifocal	Varied shapes and forms of the PVCs
Interpolated	PVC occurs during the normal R-R interval without interrupting the normal cycle
Occasional	More than one to four PVCs per minute
Frequent	More than five to seven PVCs per minute
Bigeminy	Every other beat is a PVC
Trigeminy	Every third beat is a PVC
Quadgeminy	Every fourth beat is a PVC
R on T PVCs	PVC occurs on the T wave or the vulnerable period of the ventricle refractory period
Coupling	Two PVCs occur back to back

Criteria for Classification

- *Rhythm:* The P-P and R-R intervals will be regular with early QRS complexes. Every early complex has a full compensatory pause, meaning that two R-R interval periods are required before another electrical impulse can be conducted. These two R-R intervals are placed on the beat before the early complex and evaluated with the following complex if the QRS complex falls after the second point of the calipers.
- *Rate:* The atrial and ventricular rates will be the same as for the underlying rhythm, but the early complexes will provide a faster ventricular rhythm than the normal rhythm.
- *P wave configuration:* The P wave assumes the shape of the underlying rhythm. P waves are not identified on the early ventricular complex.
- *PR interval:* The PR interval measurement follows the underlying rhythm, but in the early complex there is no P wave present.
- *QRS duration and configuration:* The QRS duration measurement follows the underlying rhythm. With the early complexes, the QRS duration must be greater than 0.12 second and will have a bizarre form. The QRS shape will have a QRS wave in one direction and a T wave going in the opposite direction.

What's Unique about Premature Ventricular Complexes?

A PVC is an early QRS complex that is wide (>0.12 second) and has a bizarre appearance. There is no P wave.

How the Patient Is Affected and What You Should Know

The clinical significance of the PVCs will depend on their frequency and the amount of decrease in cardiac output that occurs with each PVC. Since PVCs can occur in normal hearts, patients may tolerate PVCs without a noticeable change in their cardiac output and have no obvious symptoms. In fact, they may be unaware they are having PVCs. Other patients may complain of the "thump or skipping" sensation with each PVC. They may also experience dizziness and other symptoms of low cardiac output. More complex PVCs, such as frequent, multifocal, R-on-T PVCs and coupling, indicate an increased risk of developing a more serious ventricular dysrhythmia (see Table 5-5).

Observe the patient for symptoms of low cardiac output. If symptoms exist, a licensed practitioner should be notified to begin appropriate treatment. Patients are provided oxygen, since PVCs often occur because of hypoxic states (suffering from lack of oxygen). Blood samples are drawn to evaluate the hypoxic state as well as electrolyte values, specifically potassium and calcium levels.

Idioventricular Rhythm

Idioventricular rhythms occur when the sinoatrial and junctional pacemakers fail to initiate an impulse and all that is remaining is the slow ventricular pacemaker (20 to 40 beats per minute). This dysrhythmia presents with the classic "wide" QRS (0.12 second or greater), a slow ventricular rate (20 to 40), and an absence of P waves (see Figure 5-26).

Figure 5-26 Idioventricular rhythm.

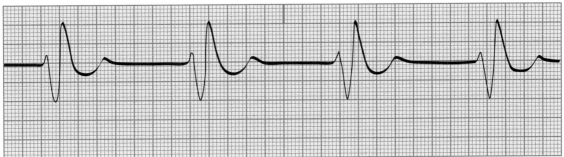

Criteria for Classification

- **Rhythm:** P-P interval cannot be determined. R-R interval is regular.
- **Rate:** Atrial rate cannot be determined due to the absence of atrial depolarization. The ventricular rate is 20 to 40 beats per minute.
- **P wave configuration:** The P wave is usually absent; therefore, no analysis of the P wave can be done.
- **PR interval:** The PR interval cannot be measured because the P wave cannot be identified.
- **QRS duration and configuration:** The QRS duration and configuration measures 0.12 second or greater and will have the classic ventricular "wide-bizarre" appearance.

What's Unique about Idioventricular Rhythm?

An idioventricular rhythm has an absence of P waves, slow ventricular rate of 20 to 40 beats per minute, and wide-bizarre QRS complexes.

How the Patient Is Affected and What You Should Know

The patient has a profound loss of cardiac output due to the loss of atrial kick and the slow ventricular rate. The patient will likely be unconscious. You must notify a licensed health care practitioner immediately. This is a medical emergency that will likely require treatment with cardiac medications and/or pacing. ECG strips obtained must be saved and mounted in the patient's medical record.

Accelerated Idioventricular Rhythm

Accelerated idioventricular rhythms occur when the sinoatrial and junctional pacemakers fail to initiate an impulse and all that is remaining is the slow ventricular pacemaker. The primary difference between accelerated idioventricular and idioventricular dysrhythmias is the heart rates. This dysrhythmia still presents with the classic "wide" QRS (0.12 second or greater) complex and an absence of P waves. The impulse rate for this dysrhythmia is 40 to 100 beats per minute. It is simply a faster idioventricular rhythm (see Figure 5.27).

Figure 5-27   Accelerated idioventricular rhythm.

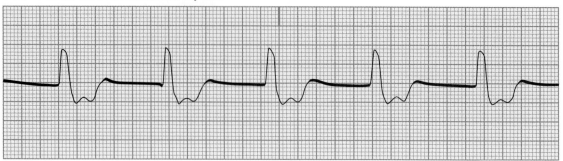

Criteria for Classification

- *Rhythm:* P-P interval cannot be determined. R-R interval is regular.
- *Rate:* Atrial rate cannot be determined due to the absence of atrial depolarization. The ventricular rate is 40 to 100 beats per minute.
- *P wave configuration:* The P wave is usually absent; therefore, no analysis of the P wave can be done.
- *PR interval:* The PR interval cannot be measured because the P wave cannot be identified.
- *QRS duration and configuration:* The QRS duration and configuration measures 0.12 second or greater and will have the classic ventricular "wide-bizarre" appearance.

What's Unique about Accelerated Idioventricular Rhythm?

The accelerated idioventricular rhythm has an absence of P waves, a ventricular rate of 40 to 100 beats per minute, and wide-bizarre QRS complexes.

How the Patient Is Affected and What You Should Know

The patient may or may not be able to tolerate this dysrhythmia due to the decrease of cardiac output as a result of the loss of atrial kick and the slower ventricular rate. The patient may or may not be unconscious. You must notify a licensed health care practitioner immediately. This patient may require treatment with cardiac medications and/or pacing. ECG strips obtained must be saved and mounted in the patient's medical record.

Ventricular Tachycardia

Ventricular tachycardia occurs when three or more PVCs occur in a row and the ventricular rate is greater than 100 beats per minute (see Figure 5-28). The ventricles are essentially in a continuous contraction-relaxation pattern and no period of delay exists between depolarization (contraction).

Criteria for Classification

- *Rhythm:* The P-P interval is usually not identifiable due to the large ventricular activity recorded. The R-R interval is usually regular, but it may be slightly irregular at times.

Figure 5-28 Ventricular tachycardia.

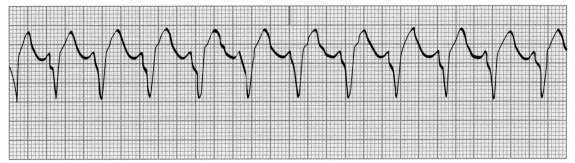

- *Rate:* Atrial rate cannot be determined because the P-P interval cannot be recognized. The ventricular rate is between 100 and 200 beats per minute.
- *P wave configuration:* The P wave is usually absent; therefore, no analysis of the P wave can be done.
- *PR interval:* The PR interval cannot be measured because the P wave is not able to be identified.
- *QRS duration and configuration:* The QRS duration and configuration measures greater than 0.12 second and will have a bizarre appearance with an increase in amplitude. The T wave will be in the opposite direction (usually downward) from that of the QRS complex.

What's Unique about Ventricular Tachycardia?

Ventricular tachycardia has a classic "sawtooth" appearance and a rate in excess of 100 beats per minute, with, no P wave.

How the Patient Is Affected and What You Should Know

The patient will have a decrease in cardiac output due to the decrease in ventricular filling time and the loss of the atrial kick. Some patients can tolerate the dysrhythmia for a short time and will have a pulse and remain conscious, whereas other patients will be unresponsive immediately. About 50% of the patients will become unconscious immediately, with no pulse or respiration.

Troubleshooting **Escape Beats**

PVCs, called "escape beats," can often occur when the heart rate is less than 60 beats per minute. This is the heart's effort to pick up the rate. The PVCs are occurring because of the bradycardia, not because of hypoxia or abnormal lab values.

Which of the following would most likely be the cause of a PVC: oxygen saturation of 89% or heart rate of 46 beats per minute?

_____

_____

Figure 5-29   Agonal rhythm.

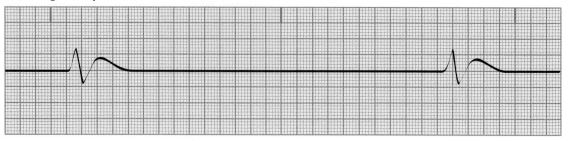

As soon as you recognize ventricular tachycardia on the monitor or ECG equipment, you should notify a licensed practitioner as the patient will need to be assessed for unresponsiveness. If the patient is unresponsive, a Code Blue is called and CPR is initiated. Emergency equipment such as a defibrillator, medications, and intubation equipment are necessary. Rhythm strips are saved to document the changes in rhythm that have occurred and should be mounted in the patient's medical record. If the patient is responsive, the licensed practitioner may initiate a treatment plan of medications and electrical treatments.

Agonal Rhythm

Agonal rhythms occur when essentially all of the pacemakers in the heart have failed. This is the last semblance of ordered electrical activity in the heart. The heart is dying. The impulses showing on the monitor are ventricular but firing at a rate of less than 20 beats per minute. This dysrhythmia presents with "wide-bizarre" QRS (0.12 second or greater) complexes, and an absence of P waves (see Figure 5-29).

Criteria for Classification

- *Rhythm:* P-P interval cannot be determined. R-R interval may or may not be regular.
- *Rate:* Atrial rate cannot be determined due to the absence of atrial depolarization. The ventricular rate is less than 20 beats per minute.
- *P wave configuration:* The P wave is absent; therefore, no analysis of the P wave can be done.
- *PR interval:* The PR interval cannot be measured because the P wave cannot be identified.
- *QRS duration and configuration:* The QRS duration and configuration measures 0.12 second or greater and will have a "wide-bizarre" appearance.

What's Unique about Agonal Rhythm?

The accelerated idioventricular rhythm has an absence of P waves, a ventricular rate of less than 20 beats per minute, and wide-bizarre QRS complexes.

Figure 5-30 Ventricular fibrillation.

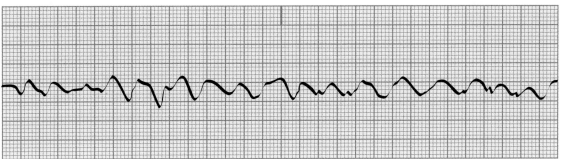

Figure 5-30 Ventricular fibrillation.

How the Patient Is Affected and What You Should Know

The patient has a profound loss of cardiac output due to the loss of atrial kick and the slow ventricular rate. The patient will be unconscious. You must notify a licensed health care practitioner immediately. This is a medical emergency that will likely require both basic life support and advanced cardiac life support interventions. ECG strips obtained must be saved and mounted in the patient's medical record.

Ventricular Fibrillation

Ventricular fibrillation is chaotic asynchronous electrical activity within the ventricular tissue. The ventricle walls are quivering, preventing any movement of blood out of the ventricles, which results in no cardiac output (see Figure 5-30). The entire myocardium is quivering similar to a bowl of Jell-O™ when shaken.

Criteria for Classification

- *Rhythm:* Both the P-P and R-R intervals cannot be determined because only chaotic waveforms are recorded on the rhythm strips. If an R-R interval is determined, it will be irregular.

- *Rate:* The atrial rate cannot be determined or identified. The ventricular rate, if identifiable, is greater than 300 beats per minute.

- *P wave configuration:* The P wave configuration is not identifiable.

- *PR interval:* The PR interval cannot be identified.

- *QRS duration and configuration:* The QRS duration and configuration cannot be determined because only fibrillatory waves are present without any uniform depolarization of the ventricle occurring.

What's Unique about Ventricular Fibrillation?

Ventricular fibrillation is the absense of organized electrical activity. The tracing is chaotic in appearance.

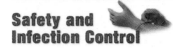

Safety and Infection Control

Crash Cart

Emergency equipment found on the "crash cart" must be ready when a code situation occurs. It is important that the cart be well stocked and the emergency equipment functioning properly. Each facility has a policy that requires regular checking and documentation of all emergency equipment and "crash carts."

How the Patient Is Affected and What You Should Know

If the patient is conscious and talking but the ECG tracing is showing ventricular fibrillation, the patient's electrodes have become loose or detached.

In true ventricular defibrillation, patients will be unresponsive when the ventricles are quivering without contracting. This will always be a Code Blue situation, in which immediate intervention is necessary to prevent biological death. Every patient experiencing ventricular fibrillation will be unconscious, apneic (**apnea** means not breathing), and pulseless. CPR and emergency measures should begin immediately. It is recommended that appropriate personnel begin the advanced cardiac life support (ACLS) to regain normal cardiac function. Rhythm strips are maintained and used as documentation in the patient's medical record.

Asystole

Asystole is absence of ventricular activity and depolarization. Often this is called "the straight or flat line" of rhythms. No electrical activity is present in the myocardium (see Figure 5-31).

Criteria for Classification

- *Rhythm:* Since no waveforms are present, there are no P-P or R-R intervals.
- *Rate:* No atrial or ventricular rates are present.
- *P wave configuration:* No P waves are present.
- *PR interval:* The PR interval is unable to be measured because no waveforms are being recorded.
- *QRS duration and configuration:* The QRS duration and configuration is not measurable because no QRS waveform is observed.

Figure 5-31 Asystole.

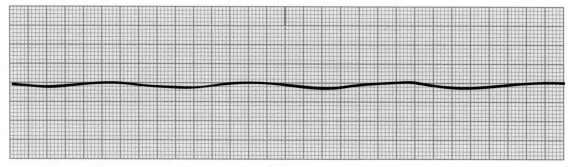

How the Patient Is Affected and What You Should Know

This rhythm is associated with life-threatening conditions. The patient will display no pulse and no cardiac output as evidenced by unconsciousness and apnea. The patient is in cardiac arrest, and emergency procedures must be initiated immediately.

Checkpoint Questions 5-9

1. What is the difference between idioventricular rhythm and accelerated idioventricular rhythm?

   _____

   _____

2. How are agonal rhythm and asystole the same?

   _____

   _____

3. What is the difference between ventricular tachycardia and ventricular fibrillation?

   _____

   _____

Answer the preceding questions and complete the "Rhythms Originating from the Ventricles" activity on the student CD under Chapter 5 before you proceed to the next section.

Patient Education & Communication

Handling Emergency Situations

During an emergency, family, friends, and other patients will be apprehensive and curious regarding the situation. You should calmly explain that there is an emergency and escort individuals out of the immediate area and view of the situation. Explain to any family members that a licensed practitioner will speak to them concerning their loved one as soon as possible.

5.10 Electronic Pacemaker Rhythms

Electronic pacemakers, also known as artificial pacemakers, are devices that deliver an electrical impulse to the myocardium to cause the cells to depolarize. This electrical generator will provide small amounts of electrical current in a predetermined interval to mimic the normal pacemaker of the heart. Pacemakers have the capability to pace the atria, ventricles, or both chambers. They are sometimes temporary but are usually implanted under the skin (see Figure 5-32) to correct dysrhythmias. Although many different types of electronic pacemakers are implanted, the mode in which they function varies in only a few ways. Because of the variety of pacemakers

Figure 5-32 Implanted pacemaker.

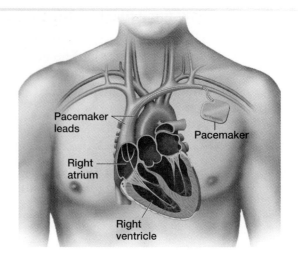

available on the market, it is recommended that you check in advance regarding the proper procedure for performing an ECG on a patient with a pacemaker.

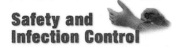

Safety and Infection Control

Pacemaker

The pacemaker's electrical current will not be dangerous to you or other people who encounter the patient. The skin does not conduct electricity so current will not be transmitted to another person from the pacemaker.

The fastest pacemaker in the heart controls the heartbeat, whether it is an inherent pacemaker, such as the SA node, or an artificial one. Electronic pacemakers work based on this principle. For example, when a patient is experiencing a bradycardia dysrhythmia, an artificial pacemaker is used and set a rate of 70 or 72 beats per minute. This artificial pacemaker will be the fastest pacemaker in the heart and thus will control the heart rate for the myocardium.

Pacemakers can stimulate several different cardiac functions. The stimulation may be for the atria, the ventricles, or both. The function will depend on the reason the pacemaker is inserted. For example, if the patient is experiencing problems with the conduction system in the ventricles, a ventricular pacemaker is inserted to deliver direct stimulation to the ventricles and produce a ventricular contraction. Atrial pacing is used alone when the conduction system from the atrioventricular node through the ventricles is intact and functioning.

Atrioventricular pacing provides direct stimulation of the atria and ventricles in a sequence pattern known as atrioventricular sequential pacing. This pacing option mimics the normal cardiac conduction system. It allows for the atria to contract completely prior to the ventricles to allow for an atrial kick. (*Remember that the atrial kick provides the extra blood supply needed for approximately 10% to 30% of the normal cardiac output.*) This pacing function is being used more when pacemakers are inserted because

Figure 5-33 The pacing spike is either atrial, ventricular, or both depending upon the type of pacemaker.

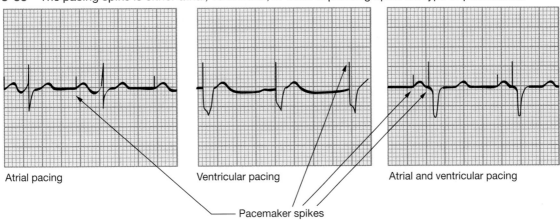

Atrial pacing

Ventricular pacing

Atrial and ventricular pacing

Pacemaker spikes

it will mimic normal cardiac function and provide the atrial kick needed. A newer type of atrioventricular sequential pacing is atriobiventricular pacing used commonly in patients with heart failure. Both ventricles are stimulated to contract compared to usually only the lower portion of the right ventricle being stimulated.

Evaluating Pacemaker Function

Pacemaker function can be evaluated based on the ECG tracings. Several different ECG characteristics must be identified prior to evaluating the pacemaker function. The most important aspect of care is to verify the effectiveness of the pacemaker and determine the presence of a pulse with each captured beat. (**Capture** refers to the ability of the heart muscle to respond to electrical stimulation and depolarize the myocardial tissue.)

Pacing Spike

The pacing spike or artifact indicates the stimulation of electrical current from the pacemaker generator. The current is a quick delivery and is reflected as a thin spike on the ECG tracing (see Figure 5-33). After the pacing spike, a tracing of either a P wave or a wide QRS complex or both will appear, depending on which chamber is being paced.

Chamber Depolarization Characteristics

If the pacemaker delivers atrial pacing, the pacing spike will be followed by a P wave. When the pacemaker delivers ventricular pacing, the pacing spike will be followed by a wide QRS complex, which looks similar to an RBBB pattern. The ventricles are stimulated low in the right ventricle, causing the myocardium to depolarize slowly. The complex is wide and shaped differently from a natural QRS complex. It is similar to the RBBB since the left ventricle takes longer than the right to depolarize because of its size.

AV Delay

The AV sequential pacemaker tracing will have an atrioventricular delay. An atrioventricular delay is similar to the measurement of the PR interval on a normal rhythm tracing. It is measured from the atrial spike to the ventricle spike. Usually this programmed time frame is somewhere between 0.12 to 0.20 second, similar to a normal PR interval.

If the patient has a normal P wave and a pacer-induced ventricular complex, the atrioventricular delay is determined from the beginning of the P wave to the ventricular spike. If the patient has a pacer-induced atrial complex and a normal QRS measurement, the measurement from the pacing spike to the beginning of the QRS complex should be less than the set atrioventricular delay time frame.

Evaluating a Pacemaker ECG Tracing

Evaluating a pacemaker rhythm involves seven steps, which are similar to those used to evaluate a nonpaced rhythm. If a patient does not have an atrioventricular sequential pacemaker, steps 3 through 5 can be eliminated. In addition, it is important to estimate the frequency of the pacemaker initiating the rhythm compared to the patient's inherent rhythm. The estimates are usually referred to in 25% intervals. If the entire rhythm strip displays an atrioventricular paced rhythm, it is referred to as 100% atrioventricular pacing (1:1). (*When less than 100% paced rhythm occurs, identify the patient's inherent rhythm and then include the estimate of paced beats and the type of pacing function as seen on the rhythm strip.*)

Step 1. *What are the rate and regularity of the paced rhythm?*

The regularity of the pacemaker spikes should be exactly the same. Only if the patient's own rhythm becomes faster than the pacemaker will the regularity be different. The rate of the pacemaker rhythm should be exactly the number at which the pacemaker was set. Often the rate is set at 70 beats per minute.

Step 2. *What are the rate and regularity of the intrinsic rhythm (the patient's own rhythm)?*

When the patient's own heart rate beats faster than the pacemaker rhythm, the patient's intrinsic rhythm will control the heart rate. The patient's own rhythm should be noted on the ECG tracing. The rate and regularity will depend on the patient's inherent rhythm.

Step 3. *Is the atrial lead sensing appropriate?* (For AV sequential pacemakers only)

The ECG tracing needs to be evaluated for the presence of atrial spikes with the P wave following the spike. Occasionally, the patient's own SA node or atrial ectopic focus will initiate atrial contraction as evidenced by a P wave without an atrial spike.

Step 4. *Is atrial capture present?* (For AV sequential and atriobiventricular pacemakers)

Every atrial spike should have a P wave after it to indicate that the electrical current is causing the cells to depolarize. The P wave after the spike indicates that the atrial capture occurred.

Step 5. *Is atrioventricular delay appropriate?* (For atrioventricular sequential and atriobiventricular pacemakers)

Measuring from the atrial spike to the ventricular spike, or from the beginning of the P wave to the ventricular spike, will give you the atrioventricular delay interval. This time frame should be the same as the atrioventricular delay set on the pacemaker program. This information should be available on the patient's medical record or pacemaker information card.

Step 6. *Is ventricular sensing appropriate?*

The ECG tracing needs to be evaluated for the presence of ventricular spikes with the wide QRS complex following the spike. Occasionally the patient's own conduction system will work appropriately, as evidenced by a normal P wave and/or QRS complex. If the ventricular contraction occurred normally before the time interval of when the pacemaker would send a ventricular impulse, the pacemaker generator will be **inhibited,** or stopped. This is evidenced by the absence of a ventricular spike.

Step 7. *Is ventricular capture present?*

Every ventricular spike should have a wide QRS complex after it to indicate that the electrical current caused the cells to depolarize. Appearance of the QRS complex after the spike indicates that ventricular capture occurred.

Pacemaker Complications Relative to the ECG Tracing

Pacemaker generators use lithium batteries to create an electrical impulse. As with any battery, the charge of the battery will decrease to the point at which the battery needs to be replaced. If a pacemaker is losing its ability to function properly, this failure will be evident on the ECG tracings. These changes in rhythms are often referred to as *complications* of the pacemaker. Complications include slower firing rates than set, less effective sensing capabilities, and lower electrical current than predetermined.

Another pacemaker complication is related to the functioning of the pacemaker generator when the sensing capability is too low. If sensing capability is low, the pacemaker will not be able to "see" the normal contractions occurring in the sensing chamber. Therefore, electrical impulses will not be inhibited but may actually be **triggered,** sending an impulse to the myocardium because the normal electrical current of the heart's conduction system was not "seen."

There are several different reasons for pacemaker complications, but only four basic dysrhythmias are evident on the ECG tracing from these complications: **malfunctioning** (failure to pace), **malsensing** (failure to sense), **loss of capture** (failure to depolarize), and **oversensing** (perceiving electrical current from sources other than the heart) (see Table 5-6).

Responsibility in caring for patients with pacemakers requires recognizing normal pacemaker rhythms and possible complications. When you are performing an ECG or monitoring a patient with a pacemaker, you should be aware of the differences in the ECG waveforms, including the

TABLE 5-6 Pacemaker Complications

Complication	Cause	What Occurs	Patient Symptoms
Malfunctioning (failure to pace)	Pacemaker does not send electrical impulse to the myocardium.	Pacemaker intervals are irregular and impulse is slower than set rate. No pacemaker spike is seen.	Patient will most often experience hypotension, lightheadedness, and blackout periods due to bradycardia conditions.
Malsensing (failure to sense)	Pacemaker does not sense the patient's own inherent rate.	May send current to heart during relaxation (repolarization) phase; also known as **pacemaker competition** with the patient's own heart	With atrial pacing, atrial fibrillation can occur; with ventricular pacing, ventricular tachycardia or ventricular fibrillation can occur.
Loss of capture (failure to depolarize)	Pacing activity occurs but myocardium is not depolarized.	Pacing spikes will occur without capture waveform such as P wave or QRS complex (see first figure).	Symptoms depend on the basic dysrhythmia and the patient's condition prior to the pacemaker insertion.
Oversensing	Pacemaker perceives electrical current from sources other than the heart.	Either (1) the patient's own heart rate is recorded and is slower than the set rate of the pacemaker or (2) the pacemaker spikes and captures at a slower rate than set (see second figure).	Patient may have signs and symptoms of low cardiac output.

Loss of capture

Oversensing

presences of a pacing spike, chamber depolarization characteristics, and an atrioventricular delay. If you observe complications of a pacemaker rhythm, immediately notify licensed personnel for appropriate treatment and interventions.

**Checkpoint
Question
5-10**

1. Name and describe four different reasons for pacemaker complications.

_____

_____

 Answer the preceding question and complete the "Electronic Pacemaker Rhythms" activity on the student CD under Chapter 5 before you proceed to the next section.

Chapter Summary

- Evaluating an ECG requires basic knowledge of the waves, segments, and intervals of the tracing and the rate, rhythm, and regularity of the heartbeat.
- The process of evaluation an ECG tracing includes determining the ECG rhythm or regularity, determining the atrial and ventricular rate, identifying the P wave configuration, measuring the PR interval, and measuring the QRS duration and analyzing the configuration.
- Sinus rhythm is effectively a normal functioning conduction system. Dysrhythmias are abnormal rhythms that indicate a problem with the electrical conduction system, including abnormal rate or regularity.
- Dysrhythmias have varied effects on the patient depending upon their severity. One common problem associated with dysrhythmias is decreased cardiac output. Decreased cardiac is indicated by pale, cool, clammy skin, low blood pressure, and other changes to the neurological, cardiac, respiratory, and urinary systems.
- Each of the dysrhythmias may affect the patient with varying degrees of severity from no changes noted by the patient, to an impending cardiac emergency. When caring for patients, you should be aware of what signs and symptoms to observe and report to your supervisor.
- Electronic or artificial pacemaker's deliver an electrical impulse that paces the atria, ventricles, or both. A pacing spike or artifact on the ECG tracing indicates the stimulation of electrical current from the pacemaker.
- Evaluating a pacemaker ECG tracing includes seven questions; what are the rate and regularity of the paced rhythm, what is the rate and regularity of the patient's own rhythm, is the atrial lead sensing appropriate, is the atrial capture present, is the AV delay appropriate, is the ventricular sensing appropriate, and is the ventricular capture present?

Chapter Review

Matching:

Match the following terms with their definitions. Place the appropriate letter on the line provided.

_____ 1. atrial kick

_____ 2. apnea

_____ 3. neurological

_____ 4. ischemia

_____ 5. vagal tone

_____ 6. syncope

_____ 7. inhibited

_____ 8. palpitations

_____ 9. supraventricular

_____ 10. J point

a. heartbeat sensation felt by the patient

b. electrical current is stopped from being sent to the myocardium

c. pertaining to the nervous system

d. patient loses consciousness

e. impulses on the vagal nerve cause inhibitory effect on the heart

f. an ectopic focus originating above the ventricles

g. point on the QRS complex at which depolarization is complete

h. absence of breathing

i. lack of oxygen to heart muscle cells

j. blood ejected into ventricles prior to ventricular systole

Multiple Choice:

Circle the correct answer.

11. What is the rate of a normal sinus rhythm?
    a. 60 to 100 beats per minute
    b. 50 to 90 beats per minute
    c. 100 to 150 beats per minute
    d. 60 to 80 beats per minute

12. What sinus rhythm has a rate of less than 60 beats per minute?
    a. Sinus tachycardia
    b. Sinus bradycardia
    c. Sinus dysrythmia
    d. Sinus rhythms

13. Which is *not* a question that needs to be answered when determining the QRS measurement?
    a. Are all the QRS complexes of equal length?
    b. What is the actual QRS measurement and is it within the normal limits?
    c. Do all QRS complexes look alike and are the unusual QRS complexes associated with an ectopic beat?
    d. Is the R-R pattern regular?

14. What sinus rhythm has a rate of more than 100 beats per minute?
    a. Sinus tachycardia
    b. Sinus bradycardia
    c. Sinus dysrhythmia
    d. Sinus rhythms

15. What rhythm shows an irregularity during inspiration and expiration?
    a. Sinus tachycardia
    b. Sinus bradycardia
    c. Sinus dysrhythmia
    d. Sinus rhythms

16. In which period of the cardiac cycle is a strong ventricular stimulus potentially dangerous?
    a. U wave
    b. P wave
    c. T wave
    d. QRS complex

17. The normal PR interval is
    a. 0.04 to 0.10 second.
    b. 0.12 to 0.20 second.
    c. 0.22 to 0.26 second.
    d. 0.28 to 0.32 second.

18. If a QRS complex is wider than 0.12 second, it most likely indicates
    a. normal ventricular conduction.
    b. delayed ventricular conduction.
    c. increased delay at the AV node.
    d. myocardial infarction.

19. What is the range of heart rate for ventricular fibrillation?
    a. 60 to 100 beats per minute
    b. 40 to 60 beats per minute
    c. 100 to 200 beats per minute
    d. Greater than 300 beats per minute

20. What is the normal, inherent rate for the AV junction?
    a. 60 to 100 beats per minute
    b. 40 to 60 beats per minute
    c. 100 to 160 beats per minute
    d. 20 to 40 beats per minute

21. Which of the following dysrhythmias is not considered part of the supraventricular tachycardia classification?
    a. Atrial fibrillation
    b. Sinus tachycardia
    c. Ventricular tachycardia
    d. Junctional tachycardia

22. What sign or symptom might a patient complain about when experiencing a supraventricular tachycardia in an unstable condition?
    a. Back pain
    b. Palpitations
    c. Hypothyroidism
    d. Chest pain and discomfort

23. The criterion needed to classify the dysrhythmia as a supraventricular tachycardia is
    a. a heart rate between 150 and 350 beats per minute.
    b. a wide QRS complex.
    c. a clear, easily identifiable P wave with the entire wave visualized.
    d. atrial and ventricular rates that are not the same.

24. What is the primary difficulty in determining a supraventricular rhythm?
    a. Determining the ventricular rate
    b. Determining the regularity
    c. Measuring the QRS interval
    d. Determining the origin of the tachycardia

25. When is the identification of the specific dysrhythmia important in terms of treatment of the patient?
    a. When the patient first complains of any signs or symptoms
    b. When the patient's heart rate has decreased to a rate of 100 to 150 beats per minute
    c. During the treatment of a fast tachycardia situation
    d. After the rhythm has been converted to a normal rhythm and/or the heart rate is between 60 and 100 beats per minute

26. You observe a wide QRS complex while continuously monitoring a patient in lead II. Which lead placement is necessary to evaluate the location of blockage in the bundle branch system?
    a. Lead I
    b. Lead V4
    c. Lead III
    d. Lead VI

27. The labeling of the ECG rhythm strip for documentation of the bundle branch block should include what other information besides which bundle is being blocked?
    a. Symptoms the patient is experiencing
    b. Blood pressure reading
    c. Presence of an MI diagnosis
    d. Patient's inherent rhythm pattern

28. What is the minimum QRS measurement for a ventricular complex?
    a. 0.06 to 0.10 second
    b. 0.04 to 0.08 second
    c. Less than 0.12 second
    d. Greater than 0.12 second

29. What do you call two PVCs that are connected to each other without a normal beat in between?
    a. Coupling or pair
    b. Run of ventricular tachycardia
    c. Frequent PVCs
    d. R-on-T PVCs

30. Which of the following is not one of the components to be evaluated on a pacemaker tracing?
    a. The presence of atrial and/or ventricular spikes
    b. The QT interval
    c. The characteristic patterns of the chambers captured after the spikes
    d. The atrioventricular delay period

Matching II

Match the following terms related to electronic (artificial) pacemakers to their definitions.

_____ 31. pacemaker competition

_____ 32. pacemaker (electronic)

_____ 33. loss of capture

_____ 34. malsensing

_____ 35. malfunctioning

_____ 36. oversensing

_____ 37. triggered

_____ 38. capture

a. electrical current causes the myocardial tissue to depolarize (contract)

b. heart muscle responds to electrical stimulation and depolarizes (contracts)

c. device that delivers electrical energy to cause depolarization (contractions)

d. pacing activity occurs but is not captured by the myocardium

e. pacemaker does not recognize the patient's inherent heart rate

f. electrical current from muscle movements or other activities are sensed by the pacemaker

g. pacemaker fails to send electrical impulse to the heart

h. patient's own heart and the electronic pacemaker compete over electrical control of the heart

What Should You Do? *Critical Thinking Application*

Read the following situations and use your critical thinking skills to determine how you would handle each. Write your answer in detail in the space provided.

39. When performing an ECG on Mr. Bobela, you notice chaotic electrical activity on the ECG tracing. Mr. Bobela was awake when you started the ECG and is lying quietly now. What should you do?

_____

_____

40. Ms. Gomez has a second degree AV block, Mobitz I rhythm. Mrs. Jenwren has a second degree AV block, Mobitz II. Which patient has a more serious condition? Explain your answer.

_____

_____

41. The rhythm on the ECG machine is ventricular tachycardia. What information would you need to know about the patient in order for proper treatment to begin?

_____

_____

42. You noticed that Mr. Green is having a wide QRS complex on the monitor. The continuous monitoring equipment has only three lead wires. How would you describe the type of block the patient is experiencing when notifying the physician of the change?

_____

_____

43. Mrs. Estes, an inpatient in your facility, has just finished shopping on the TV shopping network and knows that she has spent too much money. She is complaining that she is having palpitations. You notice that the heart rate is fast and her rhythm indicates an SVT pattern. What should you find out about the patient prior to notifying the licensed practitioner of the rapid heartbeat?

_____

_____

Rhythm Identification

Review the dysrhythmias pictured here and, using the criteria for classification provided in the chapter as clues, identify each rhythm and provide what information you used to make your decision.

44.

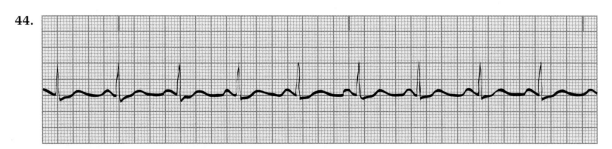

Rhythm: _____

Clues: _____

_____

_____

45.

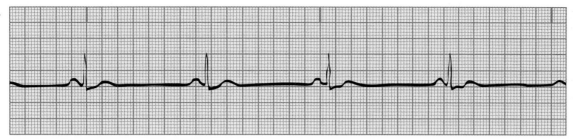

Rhythm: _____

Clues: _____

_____

_____

46.

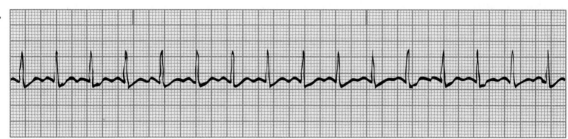

Rhythm: _____

Clues: _____

_____

_____

47.

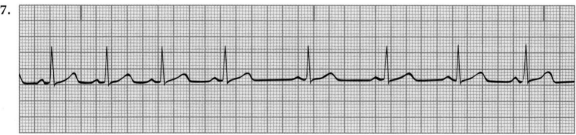

Rhythm: _____

Clues: _____

_____

_____

48.

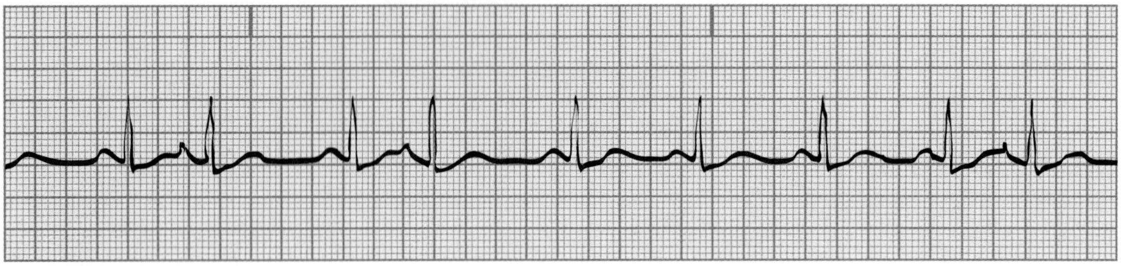

Rhythm: _____

Clues: _____

_____

_____

49.

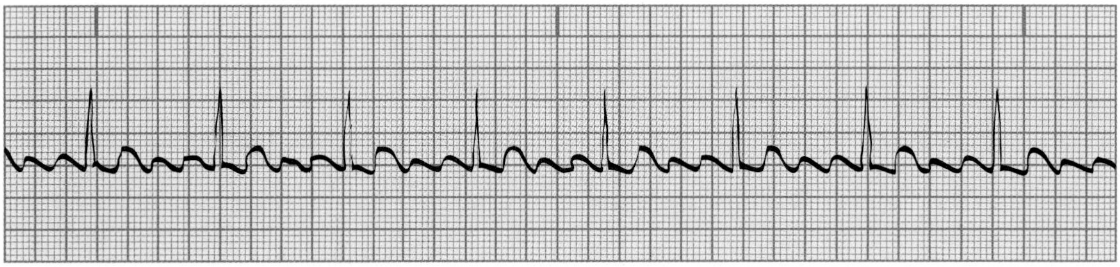

Rhythm: _____

Clues: _____

_____

_____

50.

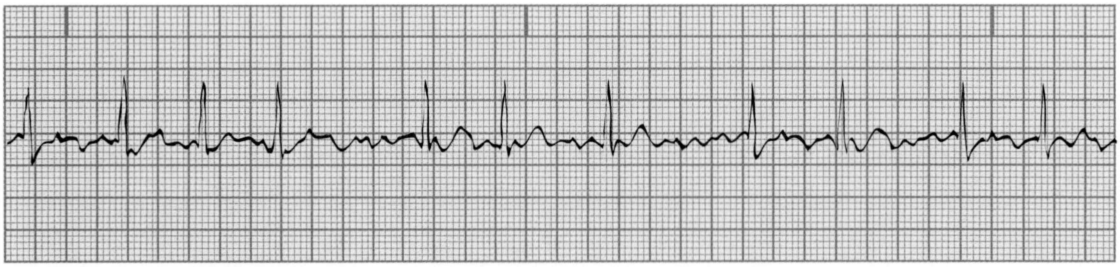

Rhythm: _____

Clues: _____

_____

_____

51.

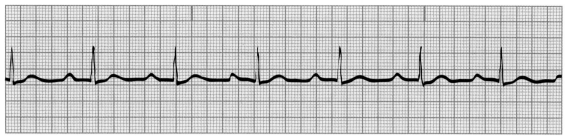

Rhythm: _____

Clues: _____

_____

_____

52.

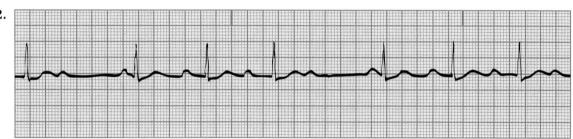

Rhythm: _____

Clues: _____

_____

_____

53.

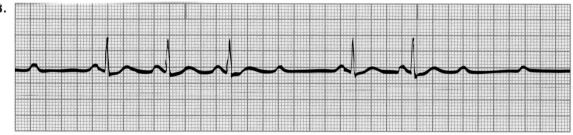

Rhythm: _____

Clues: _____

_____

_____

54.

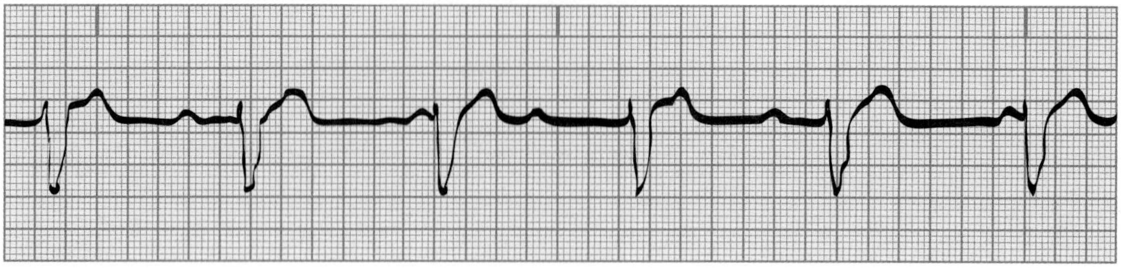

Rhythm: _____

Clues: _____

_____

_____

55.

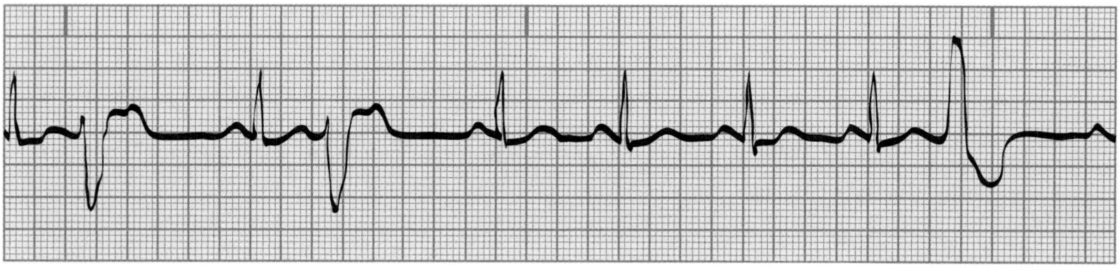

Rhythm: _____

Clues: _____

_____

_____

56.

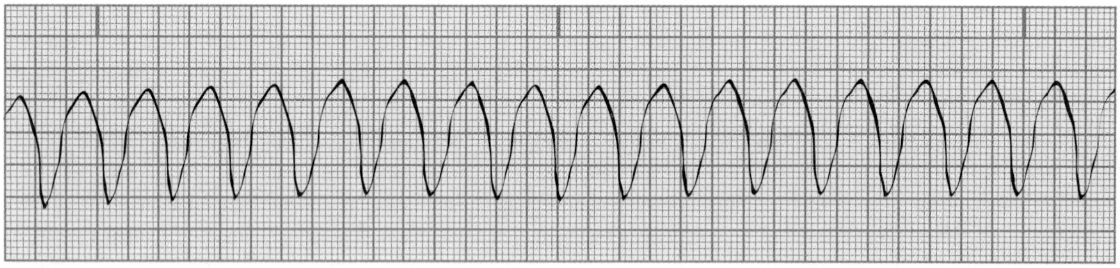

Rhythm: _____

Clues: _____

_____

_____

57.

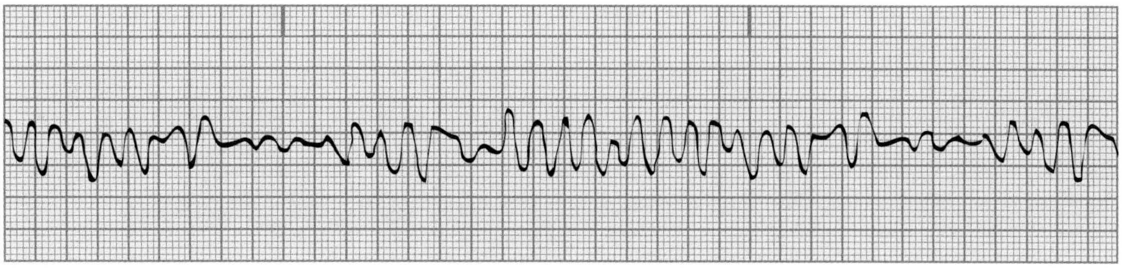

Rhythm: _____

Clues: _____

_____

_____

58

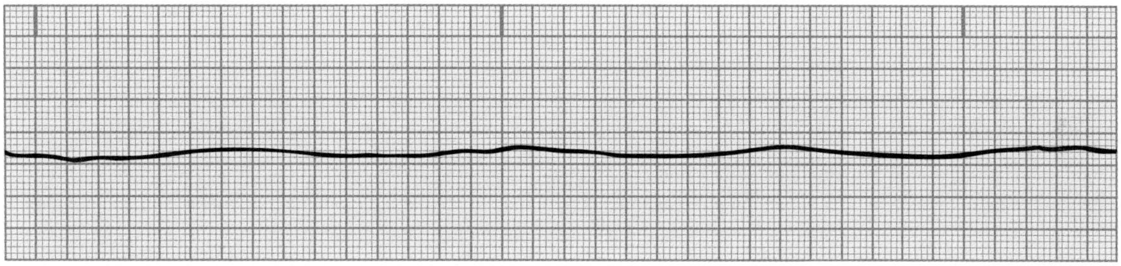

Rhythm: _____

Clues: _____

_____

_____

59.

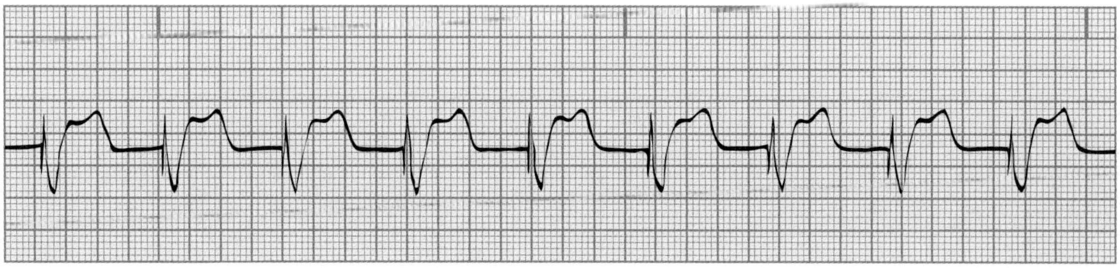

Rhythm: _____

Clues: _____

_____

_____

Perform a complete analysis of the following rhythms completing all the information in the blanks provided.

60.

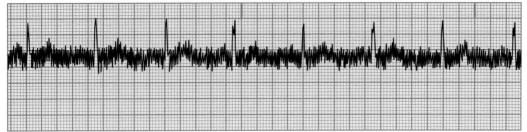

Rhythm: _____   Rate: _____

P wave: _____   PRI: _____

QRS Complex: _____   Interpretation: _____

_____

61.

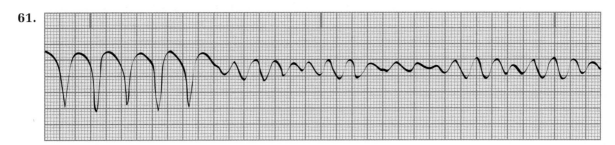

Rhythm: _____   Rate: _____

P wave: _____   PRI: _____

QRS Complex: _____   Interpretation: _____

_____

62.

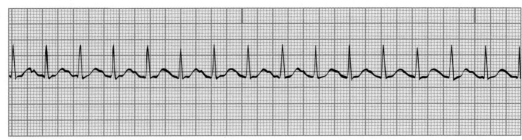

Rhythm: _____   Rate: _____

P wave: _____   PRI: _____

QRS Complex: _____   Interpretation: _____

_____

63.

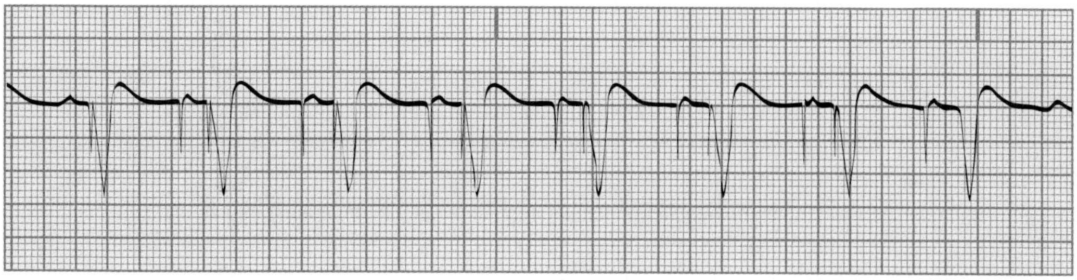

Rhythm: _____   Rate: _____

P wave: _____   PRI: _____

QRS Complex: _____   Interpretation: _____

_____

64.

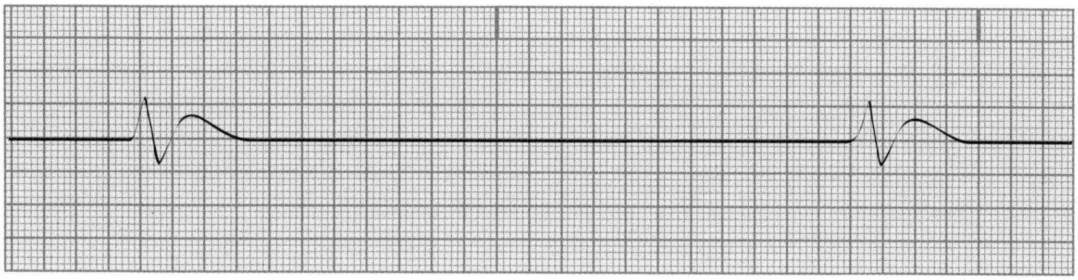

Rhythm: _____   Rate: _____

P wave: _____   PRI: _____

QRS Complex: _____   Interpretation: _____

_____

65.

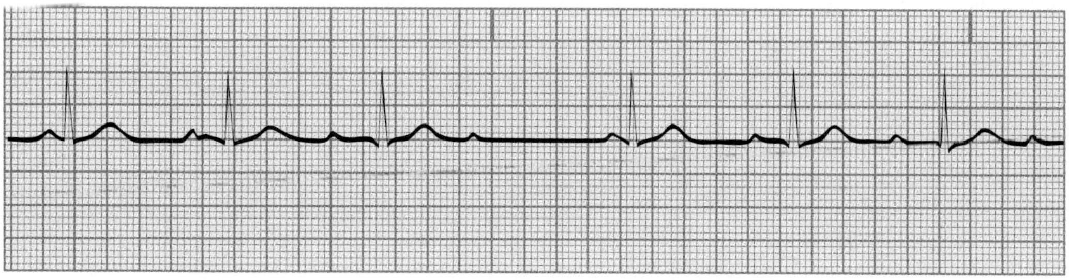

Rhythm: _____   Rate: _____

P wave: _____   PRI: _____

QRS Complex: _____   Interpretation: _____

_____

66.

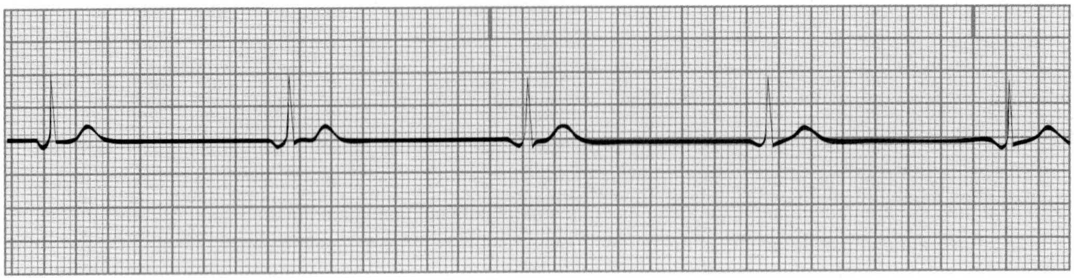

Rhythm: _____ Rate: _____

P wave: _____ PRI: _____

QRS Complex: _____ Interpretation: _____

_____

67.

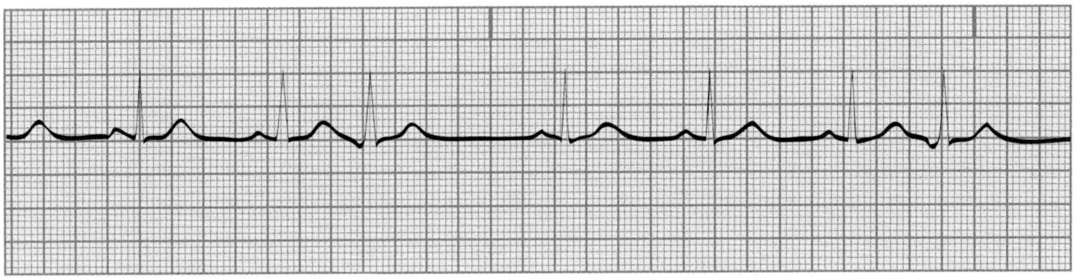

Rhythm: _____ Rate: _____

P wave: _____ PRI: _____

QRS Complex: _____ Interpretation: _____

_____

68.

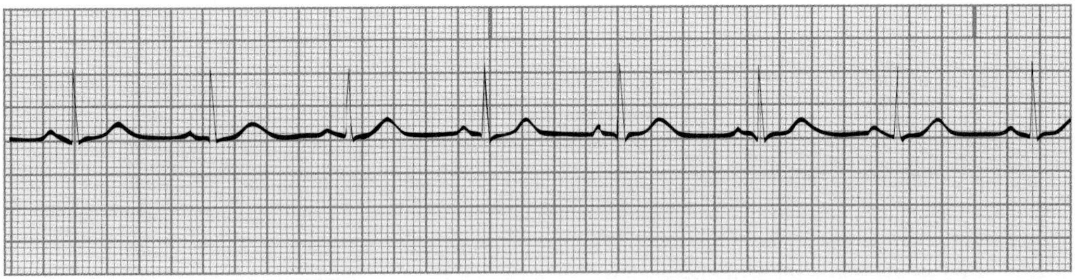

Rhythm: _____ Rate: _____

P wave: _____ PRI: _____

QRS Complex: _____ Interpretation: _____

_____

69.

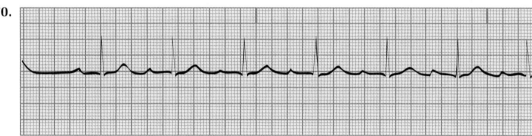

Rhythm: _____   Rate: _____

P wave: _____   PRI: _____

QRS Complex: _____   Interpretation: _____

_____

70.

Rhythm: _____   Rate: _____

P wave: _____   PRI: _____

QRS Complex: _____   Interpretation: _____

_____

71.

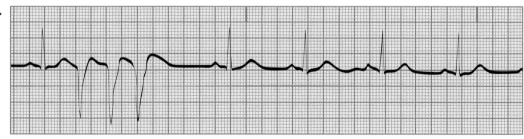

Rhythm: _____   Rate: _____

P wave: _____   PRI: _____

QRS Complex: _____   Interpretation: _____

_____

72.

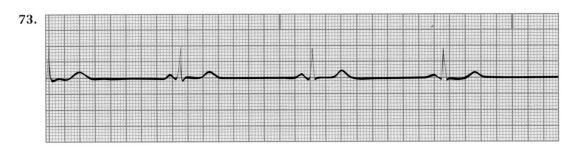

Rhythm: _____   Rate: _____

P wave: _____   PRI: _____

QRS Complex: _____   Interpretation: _____

_____

73.

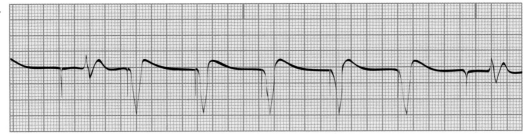

Rhythm: _____   Rate: _____

P wave: _____   PRI: _____

QRS Complex: _____   Interpretation: _____

_____

74.

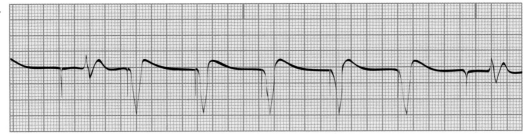

Rhythm: _____   Rate: _____

P wave: _____   PRI: _____

QRS Complex: _____   Interpretation: _____

_____

75.

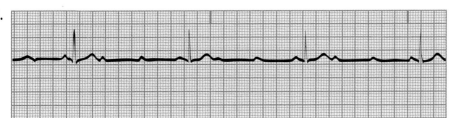

Rhythm: _____ Rate: _____

P wave: _____ PRI: _____

QRS Complex: _____ Interpretation: _____

_____

76.

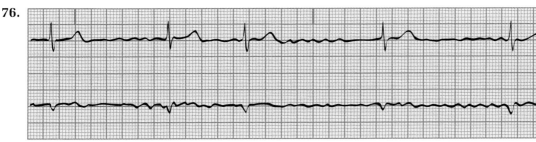

Rhythm: _____ Rate: _____

P wave: _____ PRI: _____

QRS Complex: _____ Interpretation: _____

_____

77.

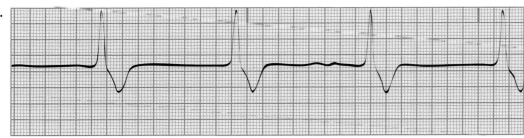

Rhythm: _____ Rate: _____

P wave: _____ PRI: _____

QRS Complex: _____ Interpretation: _____

_____

78.

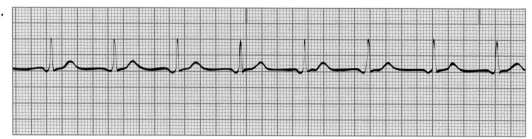

Rhythm: _____ Rate: _____

P wave: _____ PRI: _____

QRS Complex: _____ Interpretation: _____

_____

79.

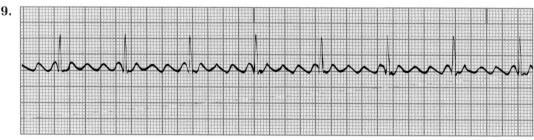

Rhythm: _____ Rate: _____

P wave: _____ PRI: _____

QRS Complex: _____ Interpretation: _____

_____

80.

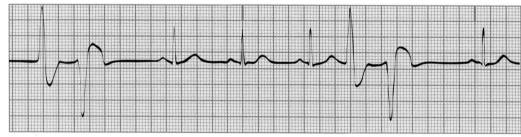

Rhythm: _____ Rate: _____

P wave: _____ PRI: _____

QRS Complex: _____ Interpretation: _____

_____

81.

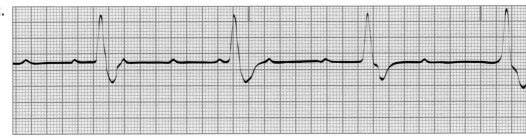

Rhythm: _____   Rate: _____

P wave: _____   PRI: _____

QRS Complex: _____   Interpretation: _____

82.

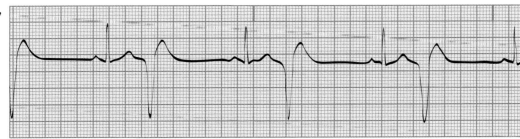

Rhythm: _____   Rate: _____

P wave: _____   PRI: _____

QRS Complex: _____   Interpretation: _____

83.

Rhythm: _____   Rate: _____

P wave: _____   PRI: _____

QRS Complex: _____   Interpretation: _____

Get Connected *Internet Activity*

Visit the McGraw-Hill Higher Education Online Learning Center *Electrocardiography for Health Care Personnel* Web site at **www.mhhe.com/healthcareskills** to complete the following activity.

1. The Alan E. Lindsay ECG Learning Center in Cyberspace is an excellent resource for more ECG learning and practice. Visit this link from the Online Learning Center and review images of rhythms, then test your knowledge. Challenge yourself and then print your scores for your instructor.

2. The 12-Lead ECG Library is also a useful site for reviewing ECGs. Go to this site from the Online Learning Center and practice before completing the rhythm identification section of this chapter.

Using the Student CD

Now that you have completed the material in the chapter text, return to the student CD and complete any chapter activities you have not yet done. Practice your terminology with the "Key Term Concentration" game. Review the chapter material with the "Spin the Wheel" game. Take the final chapter test and complete the troubleshooting question and email or print your results to document your proficiency for this chapter.

Exercise Electrocardiography

6

Chapter Outline

Learning Outcomes

- Describe exercise electrocardiography.
- Identify at least three other names for exercise electrocardiography.
- List the different uses of exercise electrocardiography.
- Describe at least one variation of exercise electrocardiography.
- Prepare a patient for exercise electrocardiography.
- Perform patient teaching for exercise electrocardiography.
- List responsibilities of a health care giver for exercise electrocardiography.
- Understand and perform proper safety measures before, during, and after exercise electrocardiography.
- Name common protocols followed in exercise electrocardiology.

Key Terms

angina	hypertension
angiogram	hyperventilate
beta blockers	invasive
cardiologist	noninvasive
congestive heart failure	skin rasp
coronary vascular disease	target heart rate (THR)
echocardiogram	thallium stress test
false positive	

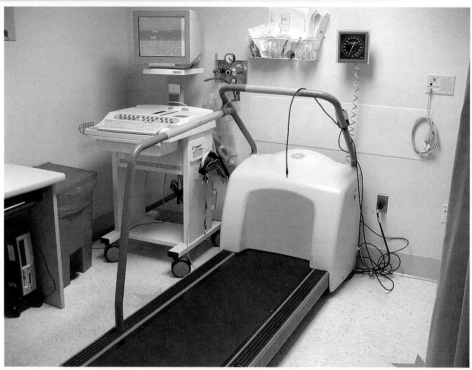

Figure 6-1 Common exercise electrocardiography equipment includes a treadmill, an ECG machine, and a monitor.

6.1 Introduction

Often a patient has symptoms of cardiac problems that do not show up on a resting ECG. In order to determine the problems and to obtain an accurate diagnosis, the physician may order an exercise electrocardiograph. Exercise electrocardiography has been used for more than 50 years. This test is known by many names, such as an exercise tolerance test, a treadmill stress test, a cardiac stress test, a stress ECG, or an exercise treadmill test. It is most commonly known as a treadmill stress test because the exercise is usually performed on an exercise treadmill (see Figure 6-1). This **noninvasive** procedure—meaning that it does not require entrance into a body cavity, tissue, or blood vessel—is an effective means of diagnosing cardiac disorders. The procedure is performed with a cardiologist or other physician present. The patient is carefully monitored throughout the testing.

Checkpoint Question 6-1

1. Why is exercise electrocardiography considered to be a noninvasive procedure?

_____

_____

6.2 What Is Exercise Electrocardiography?

During exercise electrocardiography, the patient is asked to walk on a treadmill (see Figure 6-2). While the person is exercising, his or her ECG is continuously monitored. The person is asked to increase the level of

Figure 6-2 The goal during the treadmill test is to exercise the heart and evaluate how it responds to the stress of exercise.

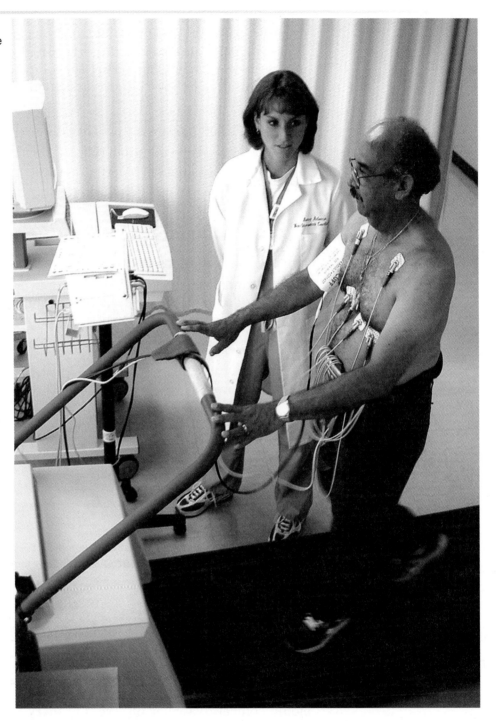

exertion of exercise as the test progresses. In addition to monitoring the ECG, the blood pressure, heart rate, skin temperature, oxygen level, and physical appearance are also assessed. Toward the end of each stage of exercise, a blood pressure and a 12-lead ECG are obtained. The patient is asked to report any chest pain, dizziness, shortness of breath, or any other symptoms. Abnormalities, physical changes, or complaints could indicate a problem that requires treatment.

As a multiskilled health care provider, you will be responsible for providing patient instructions and monitoring the patient during the procedure by taking the blood pressure, observing for pain, discomfort, fatigue, or difficulty breathing, and applying and removing the electrodes. Your most important responsibility is to provide for safety and to be prepared in case an emergency should arise. The following is a list of your responsibilities during an exercise electrocardiograph.

- Provide for safety.
- Educate and prepare the patient prior to the procedure.
- Attach the electrodes properly.
- Instruct the patient to report symptoms.
- Monitor the patient, including blood pressure and 12-lead ECG.

Patient Education & Communication

Report Abnormal Blood Pressure

Failure to report an abnormal blood pressure or other complications such as tachycardia or increased respiration rate during exercise electrocardiography could lead to severe patient problems and inaccurate test results.

Checkpoint Question 6-2

1. Name at least three responsibilities you will have during exercise electrocardiography.

   _____

   _____

 Answer the preceding question and complete the "What Is Exercise Electrocardiography?" activity on the student CD under Chapter 6 before you proceed to the next section.

6.3 Why Is Exercise Electrocardiography Used?

Exercise electrocardiography is used to evaluate how the heart and blood vessels respond to physical activity. Treadmill stress testing is typically performed when the physician suspects a cardiac problem, most commonly coronary vascular disease. **Coronary vascular disease** is usually due to atherosclerosis, which occurs when plaque forms in the blood vessels from an accumulation of excess fat. When the heart is exercised, it requires additional blood to provide oxygen to the myocardium (heart muscle). The exercise increases the myocardial oxygen demand. If a patient has narrowed or obstructed arteries due to coronary vascular disease, blood flow to the heart will not increase in response to the exercise. This additional workload may change the ECG tracing. One such change in the ECG tracing is ST segment depression, as shown in Figure 6-3. ST depression may indicate a myocardial ischemia. The exercise may also produce symptoms of chest pain (**angina**), weakness, shortness of breath, palpitations, or dizziness.

Figure 6-3 ST segment depression is depression of the ST segment below the normal baseline of the ECG. It indicates myocardial ischemia, which can occur during exercise electrocardiography.

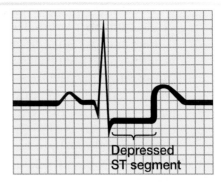

Depressed
ST segment

Exercise electrocardiography is used for other reasons as well. The physician may want to assess how well the patient's blood pressure is maintained during exercise. Exercise electrocardiography may also be used to evaluate exercise-induced symptoms such as palpitations or angina. It may also be performed to determine the patient's risk of a myocardial infarction. After an MI or cardiac surgery, the treadmill stress test is frequently used to evaluate the functioning of the heart. It may also be used to evaluate the effectiveness of cardiac medications, identify arrhythmias that occur during exercise, and aid in the development of an exercise program. The following is a list of uses for exercise electrocardiography.

- Helps diagnose cause of chest pain
- Determines functional capacity of the heart after surgery or myocardial infarction
- Screens for heart disease (particularly in men over age 35) when no symptoms are present
- Helps set limitations for an exercise program
- Identifies cause of abnormal heart rhythms that develop during physical exercise
- Evaluates effectiveness of heart medications

Checkpoint Question 6-3

1. What does exercise electrocardiography help identify?

_____

_____

Answer the preceding question and complete the "Why Is Exercise Electrocardiography Used?" activity on the student CD under Chapter 6 before you proceed to the next section.

6.4 Variations of Exercise Electrocardiography

One variation of exercise electrocardiography is a **thallium stress test.** A thallium stress test is similar to a treadmill stress test. The exercise and monitoring portion are the same; however, during a thallium stress test, the patient is injected intravenously with thallium 1 to 2 minutes before the end of the exercise period. Thallium is a radiopaque substance, which means it does not let x-rays penetrate so the thallium can be traced by an x-ray machine. Thallium flows into the heart and is viewed by the **cardiologist,** a physician who specializes in the study of the heart, using a special camera or scanner. Taking pictures of the heart lasts about 10 to 20 minutes. The patient lies on a table with both arms above the head and the scanner above them. The heart is viewed immediately after the test as well as 3 to 4 hours later, when the patient has rested. The cardiologist studies the pictures to determine if blood flow to the heart improves with rest. Thallium flows more easily through nondiseased arteries. The purpose of the procedure is to determine if exercise causes a decrease in blood flow to any area of the heart. This procedure is considered **invasive** since the patient is injected with thallium.

Patient Education & Communication

Complete Explanation Is Necessary

Patient education brochures are valuable to help the patient understand the procedure. However, they may not be enough. The physician should explain the purpose for the test, but it is your responsibility to ensure that the patient understands what will occur during the test and what the patient should report to the physician while the test is in progress.

Another variation of the exercise electrocardiography is a Persantine-thallium stress test. This test is similar to a thallium stress test with one exception: it is performed on patients who are not able to exercise. During this test, the physician or nurse administers medication called Persantine® (dipyridamole), which causes the heart to exercise artificially. The medication is injected over time to stimulate the heart to exercise throughout the testing. When Persantine and thallium are used in combination, this is known as a Persantine-thallium stress test. This test requires the patient to have intravenous injections of both thallium and Persantine.

Checkpoint Question 6-4

1. Why would it be necessary to use chemical stress testing?

_____

_____

 Answer the preceding question and complete the "Variations of Exercise Electrocardiography" activity on the student CD under Chapter 6 before you proceed to the next section.

6.5 Preparing and Educating the Patient

When scheduling a patient for exercise electrocardiography, you will need to make sure the patient comes prepared for the test (see Table 6-1, "The Stress Test Procedure"). Describe the procedure and ensure that the patient

TABLE 6-1   The Stress Test Procedure

When Setting the Appointment

- Verify that the medical history is complete.
- Explain the procedure, including the reason for test, possible complications, and *safety* measures that will be followed during procedure.
- Explain "Informed Consent" and ask the patient to sign consent form.
- Inform patients that the day of the test they should wear comfortable clothing (shorts, tennis shoes, etc.). Female patients should not wear an underwire bra. Refrain from use of tobacco, caffeine, or alcohol for *at least 3 hours* prior to test. The patient should eat a light meal 2 hours prior to the test.
- Check the physician's orders against the patient medication list to provide information as to what medications the patient should *not* take the day of the test.
- Go over all instructions and information with the patient. Encourage questions; make sure the patient fully understands the procedure.
- Provide a detailed list of instructions making sure that your facility telephone number and your name appear on the list. Encourage patients to call if they have any questions prior to test day.

Day of Appointment

- Verify that equipment is in working order and supplies are on hand. (Ensure plenty of tracing paper, inspect cables, check that treadmill is working, and verify computer setup and correct protocol.)
- Gather supplies—electrodes, alcohol, gauze sponges, razor, adhesive tape, blood pressure cuff, and so on.
- Check that the *crash cart* is ready and fully supplied and the defibrillator is working.
- Verify the physician's order, that the medical history is complete, and that the informed consent is signed.
- Bring the patient into the room.
- Verify with the patient that he or she has complied with all instructions.
- Provide the patient with privacy to change into gown with the opening to the front unless the patient needs assistance. Female patients should not wear an underwire bra.
- *Remember: During all aspects of the procedure, always provide for safety of the patient!*
- Assist the patient to lie down on the table. Prep the patient's skin and apply electrodes as indicated by the protocol of the facility or the equipment manual.
- Connect cables, apply the blood pressure cuff, and check the ECG tracing for artifact.
- Obtain the patient's blood pressure and ECG in the following positions (assist the patient as necessary and provide for safety):
  - Supine
  - Sitting
  - Sitting, post 30-second hyperventilation
  - Standing

  (Make sure you change the resting position in the stress test machine and enter a new blood pressure for each tracing.)
- Demonstrate the treadmill (posture, hand grip, etc.).
- Explain the test protocol, making sure the patient understands that the speed and incline will increase every 3 minutes during the test phase.
- *Be sure the patient understands that he or she is to report any pain, shortness of breath, faintness, tingling sensations, numbness, or extreme fatigue immediately! Monitor patient closely during the test looking for visual signs of any of the above. Ask the patient repeatedly during the procedure how he or she feels. Providing for patient safety is your number one priority!*
- Explain again that the test will be completed when the target heart rate is reached [(220 – age) × 0.85] or when the patient cannot continue due to fatigue or other symptoms.
- Inform the physician that the patient is ready to begin the test. The physician should be present and immediately available.
- When the physician is in the room, assist the patient to the treadmill, making sure the patient's feet are not on the belt. Start the belt; tell patient to get used to the speed and then to step onto the belt. Ask the patient if he or she is ready to begin, explaining again that the belt speed and incline will increase. Begin the test phase.

(Continued)

- At the 2½-minute mark of each phase, take the patient's blood pressure and enter the data into the computer. Remind the patient before every transition to a new phase. *Be ready* to assist the patient as needed.
- When the treadmill phase of the test is complete (the target heart rate is reached or the patient cannot continue), assist the patient to a waiting chair.

Posttest
- Continue to monitor and observe the patient's condition closely, taking the patient's blood pressure, entering data, and then taking an ECG tracing every 3 to 5 minutes for 10 to 15 minutes.
- When the cooldown period is completed, remove the cables and electrodes; wipe off any remaining gel or adhesive.
- Allow the patient to dress (assist if needed).
- Explain to the patient that he or she should avoid tobacco, caffeine, and alcohol for at least 3 hours. The patient should avoid extreme temperature changes, including hot showers or baths for 2 hours. The patient should rest and recuperate after the test.
- Explain that the physician will have the results of the test in 10 days. Thank the patient for his or her participation.
- File your report per the protocol of the facility.
- Make sure all information from the patient chart is returned to its proper place.
- Prepare for the next patient.

understands. The patient should not smoke or drink alcohol or caffeine 3 hours prior to the test. He or she should also be advised not to eat for at least 2 hours before the test. The patient should be instructed to bring or wear comfortable clothing and shoes. Tennis shoes and loose pants will make the exercise portion of the test easier for the patient.

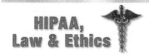
HIPAA, Law & Ethics

Informed Consent

Informed consent is required for surgery, HIV testing, and other procedures, including exercise electrocardiography. Informed consent implies that the patient understands the treatment, why it is being performed, any risks to the patient, alternative treatments and their risks, and the risk involved if the patient refuses treatment. Listed in Table 6-2 are typical reasons patients refuse the test and suggestions for resolving the problem.

What happens when you ask the patient to sign an informed consent form and he or she refuses?

_____

_____

Sometimes certain medications should not be taken prior to the test. You will need to instruct the patient regarding medications that should or should not be taken. Always check the physician's order. If it is not written on the chart or order, ask the physician. When asking, have a list of the patient's current medications or the patient's chart available for the physician to review. Medications commonly known as **beta blockers**—drugs used to treat hypertension—are frequently stopped prior to an exercise electrocardiography test because this type of medication could affect the test

TABLE 6-2 Handling a Patient's Refusal to Grant Consent

Reason for Refusal	Possible Solution
Patient does not understand why the consent form is necessary.	Explain the legal requirement of an informed consent and refer the patient to the physician for questions, if necessary.
Patient does not understand the procedure.	Notify the physician and provide a brochure for the patient to review while he or she is waiting for the physician to explain the procedure.
Patient is illiterate and unable to sign his or her name.	Have a witness present (preferably a family member) and have the consent form marked with an X by the patient and signed by the witness and yourself.
Patient is unable to sign because glasses are not available.	Make every attempt to obtain the glasses and then have the patient sign; if this is not possible, have the patient sign to the best of his or her ability; be certain to have a witness (preferably a family member) sign the form as well.

results or delay the test. See Appendix for more information about common cardiovascular medications. Remember, your responsibility is to ensure that the patient comes to the office or clinic properly prepared for the exercise electrocardiography test.

A complete history of the patient may need to be recorded before beginning the test. A standard form should be used. The information you need to obtain from the patient includes the medical history, medications currently being taken, cardiovascular risk factors (see Table 1-1 in Chapter 1), and the reason for this examination. Much of this information may already be on the patient's chart. In addition, an informed consent form must be signed and witnessed (see Figure 6-4). The patient should understand the procedure, its risks, and the reason the test has been ordered before signing the informed consent form.

The patient should be informed that exercise electrocardiography is not a "timed" test. The length of time the test takes depends on several factors, including the patient's age, degree of conditioning or health status, other medical problems, and medications. You should inform the patient that the test will take approximately 45 minutes to an hour. Carefully explain the safety precautions provided during the procedure to help alleviate any fears the patient may have.

Checkpoint Question 6-5

1. Stress testing is a noninvasive procedure. Why is informed consent necessary?

_____

_____

 Answer the preceding question and complete the "Preparing and Educating the Patient" activity on the student CD under Chapter 6 before you proceed to the next section.

Figure 6-4 Your patient must sign an informed consent for exercise electrocardiography. Most facilities use a standardized form such as the one pictured here.

Consent Form for Exercise/Chemical Stress Testing

A Stress Test is being performed to provide information about the blood supply to your heart, as well as to assess your ability to do various activities.

In order to determine an appropriate plan of medical management, I hereby consent to voluntarily engage in a myocardial stress test to determine the state of my heart and circulation.

The information obtained will help my physician recommend treatment options regarding my cardiovascular health. The test that I will undergo will be performed on a treadmill with the amount of effort increasing gradually as the test progresses. This increase in effort will continue until either a predetermined heart rate is achieved or symptoms such as fatigue, shortness of breath, or chest discomfort appear, which indicate to me to stop. An alternative type of stress test may be administered where a medication may be used to "stress" or exercise the heart. During the performance of the test, trained staff will closely monitor my pulse, blood pressure, and electrocardiogram.

If performed as part of a nuclear myocardial perfusion study, I will be injected with a small amount of radioactive material (Thallium) followed by imaging of the heart. The amount of radioactivity I will be exposed to is about equivalent to a chest x-ray.
There is always the possibility of certain changes occurring during the test. They include abnormal blood pressure, fainting, shortness of breath, abnormal heart rhythms (too rapid, too slow, or ineffective), and very rare instances of heart attack. Every effort will be made to minimize them by the preliminary examination and by observations during and immediately after testing. Emergency equipment and highly trained personnel are available to manage any unusual situations that may arise.

I have read the above information and understand the procedures, as well as any possible complications or risks. I understand that in rare instances, heart attack or stroke has been reported. I acknowledge that my physician has explained my condition and the nature and purpose of this test, as well as alternative tests, and that all questions asked about my care and its attendant risks have been answered in a satisfactory manner. I understand that any question(s) I still may have can be answered by my physician or clinic staff members at any time. I hereby accept the risk of harm, if any, in hopes of obtaining the desired beneficial diagnostic information.

Signed:

_____   _____
Patient   Date

_____   _____
Patient Name Printed   Witness

_____
Physician Supervising Test

6.6 Providing Safety

Exercise electrocardiography is done on patients who are already at risk. At-risk patients may have just recently had a myocardial infarction or may currently be experiencing some type of chest pain or other symptoms, or they may have a history of coronary vascular disease. Exercise electrocardiography does place stress on the patient's heart. There is some risk of a heart attack or stroke during the procedure that should be considered. You should follow the safety measures and be prepared for emergencies (see Table 6-3).

In order to provide for safety, certain rules must be followed. A physician should always be present during the procedure. Emergency equipment

- Inform the patient how he or she can expect to feel during the test, including mild fatigue, increased heart rate, perspiration, and increased breath rate.

- Explain to the patient the need to report signs and symptoms such as chest or other pain, dizziness, weakness, or extreme fatigue.

- Make sure the patient knows to stop the exercise if any pain or extreme fatigue is felt.

- *Make sure the physician is present during the entire procedure.*

- Check to see that emergency equipment is close by, including a code or crash cart with defibrillator

- Observe and monitor the patient and report any symptoms to the physician.

should be in the room or nearby, including a crash cart with emergency medications and supplies. You must know the location of this equipment. In addition, the patient should be monitored at all times and he or she must understand the need to report any abnormal symptoms when they occur.

Some health conditions prevent patients from participating in exercise electrocardiography. These conditions include but are not limited to

- Heart aneurysm
- Uncontrolled disturbances in the heartbeat
- Inflammation surrounding the heart or heart muscle
- Severe anemia
- Uncontrolled **hypertension** (high blood pressure)
- Unstable angina
- **Congestive heart failure** (the heart's failure to pump an adequate volume of blood)

The physician should be aware of any of these conditions. Make sure that the health history is current and complete for the physician to review.

Checkpoint Question 6-6

1. Can everyone have a standard stress test? What are some reasons why not?

_____

_____

 Answer the preceding question and complete the "Providing Safety" activity on the student CD under Chapter 6 before you proceed to the next section.

6.7 Performing Exercise Electrocardiography

Assemble and prepare the equipment before the patient's arrival. You will need

- Blood pressure equipment
- Shaving equipment, abrasive skin cleaner, skin rasp

CPR Required

As a multiskilled health care provider, you should know cardiopulmonary resuscitation (CPR) and be prepared to respond to cardiac or respiratory emergencies.

- Alcohol solution
- 2 × 2 or 4 × 4 gauze
- Chest electrodes
- Stress test unit
- Lead wires
- Treadmill or stationary bicycle
- Adhesive tape belt (used to attach monitoring unit) or mesh vest

When the patient arrives for the test, you should verify that he or she has come properly prepared by making sure the patient has not had alcohol, caffeine, or tobacco for at least 3 hours or food for 2 hours prior to the test. Verify that medications were stopped, if required. Complete the patient's medical history and make sure the informed consent form has been signed.

Next, prepare the electrode sites for placement. If the sites are hairy, dry shave the skin. Rub the site with an alcohol swab and let it dry. Abrade the skin using a special prep pad, dry 4 × 4 gauze, **skin rasp,** or other type of abrasive cleaner. Abrading the skin consists of rubbing firmly and briskly at each of the sites where the electrodes will be placed to ensure that they will adhere better to the skin.

Attach the blood pressure cuff and electrodes. Check the manufacturer's instructions for the system you are using and the policy at your facility for correct placement of the electrodes (see Figure 6-5). Some machines include a diagram that provides information for correct placement (see Figure 6-6). Many exercise electrocardiography monitors include leads for both chest and back.

Troubleshooting

Reporting Problems

If your patient has any complaints or problems during exercise electrocardiography, you should be prepared to respond. Keep in mind that while the physician should be in the room, he or she may not always be aware of the patient's complaints or problems. Any symptom that the patient reports such as extreme fatigue, dizziness, shortness of breath, or chest pain should be immediately reported to the physician.

What should you do if the patient collapses?

_____

_____

Prior to the exercise test, a series of blood pressures and 12-lead ECGs will be obtained with the patient in different positions. The following is a

Figure 6-5 Standard placement of electrodes for exercise electrocardiography is usually the same as a 12-lead ECG. Since machines may vary, check the manufacturer's instructions for proper placement of the electrodes for the exercise electrocardiograph machine you are using.

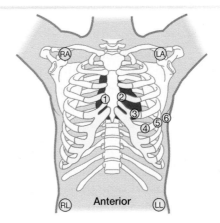

common example. Your facility may or may not use each of these pretest steps. Check the policy where you are employed.

First: A resting ECG and blood pressure are obtained while the patient is supine.

Second: The patient is asked to sit up and another blood pressure and ECG are obtained.

Third: The patient is asked to breathe quickly and deeply (**hyperventilate**) for about 30 seconds. Then another blood pressure and ECG are taken. This ECG is done to identify ECG changes caused by breathing. These changes could be misinterpreted as being related to heart disease if they occurred during the stress test.

Fourth: The patient is asked to stand and the final preexercise blood pressure and ECG are obtained.

Figure 6-6 Diagram found on one type of exercise electrooardiograph machine showing proper electrode placement.

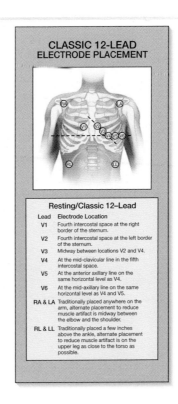

CLASSIC 12-LEAD
ELECTRODE PLACEMENT

Resting/Classic 12–Lead

Lead	Electrode Location
V1	Fourth intercostal space at the right border of the sternum.
V2	Fourth intercostal space at the left border of the sternum.
V3	Midway between locations V2 and V4.
V4	At the mid-clavicular line in the fifth intercostal space.
V5	At the anterior axillary line on the same horizontal level as V4.
V6	At the mid-axillary line on the same horizontal level as V4 and V5.
RA & LA	Traditionally placed anywhere on the arm, alternate placement to reduce muscle artifact is midway between the elbow and the shoulder.
RL & LL	Traditionally placed a few inches above the ankle, alternate placement to reduce muscle artifact is on the upper leg as close to the torso as possible.

Observe Patients Carefully

Observe your patient carefully when he or she changes position and during hyperventilation for dizziness and potential for a syncopal (fainting) episode. Many of your patients will have cardiac and/or vascular disease that increases the chances for these symptoms.

The test is divided into stages of 2 or 3 minutes each. Each stage is based upon stress test protocols. The protocols include the length of time of exercise and the incline of the treadmill. The physician determines the protocol or length and incline of each stage of exercise (see Table 6-4, "Common Stress Testing Protocols"). The entire exercise period lasts up to 15 minutes. The time may vary based on the patient's cardiac risk factors and ability. Toward the end of each stage, the patient's blood pressure is checked, the ECG is repeated, and the level of exercise is increased.

TABLE 6-4 Common Stress Testing Protocols

Bruce Protocol: Most commonly utilized stress test 3-minute stages

Stage	Speed (mph)	Grade (%)
1	1.7	10
2	2.5	12
3	3.4	14
4	4.2	16
5	5.0	18
6	5.5	20
7	6.0	22

"Modified" Bruce Protocol: Most often used in older individuals or those whose exercise capacity is limited by cardiac disease 3-minute stages

Stage	Speed (mph)	Grade (%)
1	1.7	0
2	1.7	5
3	1.7	10
4	2.5	12
5	3.4	14
6	4.2	16
7	5.0	18
8	5.5	20

(Continued)

Naughton Protocol: Better suited for sicker patients, more gradual increase in intensity. Speed stays at 2 mph. Stage time is 2 minutes.

Stage	Grade (%)
1	0.0
2	3.5
3	7.0
4	10.5
5	14.0
6	17.5
7	21.0

Most people exercise to the point of fatigue or symptoms of chest discomfort or shortness of breath. The supervising physician may halt the test because of blood pressure, ECG, or heart rhythm changes that are not perceived by the patient. In other words, though the patient may not complain of any symptoms, the physician may identify changes in the blood pressure, heart rate, or ECG tracing that may lead to complications and may order that the test be stopped.

Patient Education & Communication

Reducing the Patients Fears

You can help reduce the patient's fears by maintaining a sense of confidence, answering questions, and following safety precautions during exercise electrocardiography.

During the test, the goal is to achieve the **target heart rate** (THR) without symptoms or complications. The target heart rate is 220 minus the patient's age times a percentage that ranges between 60 and 85 depending upon which testing protocol is being followed (often referred to as *submaximal exercise*). This is different from the target heart rate for aerobic exercise, which is simply 220 minus the age of the person without using an additional multiplier (often referred to as *maximal exercise*).

The THR is the rate that the patient should not be allowed to exceed during the test. Achieving the THR without symptoms or abnormalities is a good indication that the heart is functioning well. Generally, the closer the patient is to the target heart rate, the more reliable the test results.

Instruct the patient to report any symptoms such as shortness of breath, chest pain, dizziness, or weakness he or she experiences during the procedure because you are responsible for monitoring and recording this information. You will need to monitor blood pressure, pulse, and any signs of cardiac distress. You may also be monitoring the patient's blood oxygen level on the monitor screen.

Rate pressure product (RPP) or double product is a measurement that may be asked for by the doctor. It is as simple as multiplying the systolic blood pressure times the patient's heart rate. This is one technique used to estimate oxygen utilization or myocardial work. For example:

$$\text{Systolic blood pressure (SYS BP)} = 118$$

$$\text{Heart rate (HR)} = 88$$

$$\text{SYS BP} \times \text{HR} = \text{RPP}$$

$$118 \times 88 = \text{RPP}$$

$$10{,}384 = \text{RPP}$$

Watch the patient closely including skin color, breathing pattern, amount of perspiration, and facial expressions. Many times a patient is hesitant to report a symptom. If you suspect a problem, ask the patient and then report your suspicion to the supervising physician.

Checkpoint Question 6-7

1. What is the target heart rate of a patient who is 49 years old?

_____

_____

 Answer the preceding question and complete the "Performing Exercise Electrocardiography" activity on the student CD under Chapter 6 before you proceed to the next section.

6.8 Following Exercise Electrocardiography

When the patient has completed the exercise portion of the test, monitoring will continue during a "cooling off" period. This will last approximately 10 to 15 minutes. You will need to stay with the patient and continue to monitor the patient for any changes.

Many factors are used to interpret the results of exercise electrocardiography. The most important factors are the presence of ECG changes and symptoms. Other factors include heart rate and rhythm, blood pressure, and changes in oxygen consumption. If a patient has no abnormal ECG changes or unusual elevations in blood pressure, this usually means the risk for coronary vascular disease is low. If the test is stopped early because of ECG or blood pressure changes or patient symptoms, this is a sign of abnormal test results. When the results of the test are inconclusive or abnormal, additional tests may be performed. An inconclusive test is one with questionable results, meaning it does not necessarily show an abnormality or eliminate the potential for an abnormality. Additional testing is needed to either identify or eliminate any abnormalities. These additional tests may include an **echocardiogram,** which uses sound to study the heart and blood vessels (also known as ultrasound), or a coronary **angiogram,** involving x-rays following injection of a radiopaque substance.

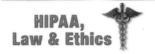
After exercise electrocardiography, the patient should be given some instructions. These include the following:

- Rest for several hours.
- Avoid extreme temperature changes.
- Avoid stimulants, such as caffeine, tobacco, or alcohol, for at least 3 hours.
- Do not take a hot shower or bath for at least 2 hours.
- Do not expect results of the examination for up to 10 days; discuss the results with your physician when available.

Stress testing is considered a good method to detect early coronary artery disease and delay its progression. However, it is interesting to note that approximately 5% of healthy adults may have **false positive** results, meaning that the test may indicate that disease is present when it is not. Research has shown that false positives occur more frequently in females than in males, though researchers are not sure why. False positives can cause unnecessary fears and the need for additional expensive tests.

Checkpoint Question 6-8

1. Name at least three instructions you would give a patient after exercise electrocardiograpy.

   _____

   _____

 Answer the preceding question and complete the "Following Exercise Electrocardiography" activity on the student CD under Chapter 6 before you proceed to the next section.

Chapter Summary

- Exercise electrocardiography is the recording of an ECG and monitoring of a patient during active or medication-induced exercise to diagnose problems that do not occur when the patient is at rest.
- Exercise electrocardiography is also known as an exercise tolerance test, treadmill stress test, a cardiac stress test, a stress ECG, or an exercise treadmill test.
- Exercise electrocardiography is used to diagnose the cause of chest pain, determine the capacity of the heart, screen for heart disease, set limits for exercise, identify abnormal heart rhythms, and evaluate the effectiveness of heart medications.
- The thallium and the Persantine thallium stress tests are variations of exercise electrocardiography that include the injection of medications before the procedure.
- To prepare a patient for exercise electrocardiography you must schedule the appointment, educate the patient, obtain a consent form, and document what you have completed.
- Prior to exercise electrocardiography the patient needs to be taught about the procedure, its complications, what to wear, what medications or other substances they can and cannot take, and what to report during the procedure itself.
- As an assistant during the procedure you may be responsible for safety, education and preparation of the patient, attachment of the electrodes, instructions on reporting symptoms, and monitoring the patient including taking the blood pressure.
- Providing for safety before, during, and after exercise electrocardiography includes following standard precautions, preparing the crash cart, monitoring the patient, providing complete patient instructions, and making sure the physician is present during the entire exercise portion of the procedure.
- Common protocols for the exercise electrocardiography include Bruce, Modified Bruce, and Naughton.

Chapter Review

Multiple Choice:

Circle the correct answer for each of the following.

1. What is your most important responsibility during exercise electrocardiography?
   a. Providing for safety
   b. Applying the leads
   c. Monitoring the ECG tracing
   d. Taking the patient's blood pressure

2. Which of the following conditions would be a reason that a patient should not perform exercise electrocardiography?
   a. Coronary vascular disease
   b. Previous heart attack
   c. Congestive heart failure
   d. Previous symptoms of angina

3. What type of test would be performed on a patient who is unable to stand or exercise?
   a. Thallium stress test
   b. Persantine-thallium test
   c. Treadmill stress test
   d. Cardiac stress test

4. During exercise electrocardiography, your patient appears to be short of breath. After informing the physician of your suspicions, what would you do?
   a. Continue the test.
   b. Take the patient's blood pressure.
   c. Ask the patient to stop the exercise portion of the test.
   d. Without the patient's knowledge, count the respiratory rate and compare to the previous rate.

5. Mr. Jones is on several medications and is scheduled for an exercise electrocardiography test tomorrow. What should you do first to determine if he should take his medications prior to the test?
   a. Check the chart or order.
   b. Ask the physician.
   c. Instruct the patient not to take his beta blocker medications.
   d. Mr. Jones should take all of his medications since they are necessary for his treatment.

6. A beta blocker is
   a. a protocol for exercise electrocardiography.
   b. a medication for hypertension.
   c. necessary when performing exercise electrocardiography.
   d. a medication for heart disease.

7. Which of the following is measured during exercise electrocardiography?
   a. Blood pressure and temperature
   b. Blood pressure and weight
   c. 12-lead ECG and weight
   d. 12-lead ECG and blood pressure

8. When educating the female patient for exercise electrocardiography, you should instruct her *not* to wear
   a. shorts.
   b. tennis shoes.
   c. an underwire bra.
   d. comfortable clothing.

Patient Education:

You are assigned to teach Mr. Hussein about exercise electrocardiography. From the following list, determine which are correct patient instructions for exercise electrocardiography and which are not. Place a *C* beside the correct statements and an *I* beside the incorrect statements. For each of the incorrect (*I*) statements, write the correct instructions for the patient.

_____ 9. Patients should avoid alcohol, tobacco, and caffeine for at least 8 hours prior to exercise electrocardiography.

_____

_____

_____ 10. Patients should be encouraged to report any symptoms such as shortness of breath, weakness, dizziness, or fatigue during exercise electrocardiography.

_____

_____

_____ 11. After exercise electrocardiography, the patient should not take a hot bath or shower for at least 2 hours.

_____

_____

_____ 12. You should discuss the results of exercise electrocardiography with the patient as soon as the results are available.

_____

_____

_____ 13. Patients should wear comfortable, casual clothing on the day of the test including tennis shoes and loose fitting pants.

_____

_____

_____ 14. You should attach the leads to the chest at the same sites as you would for an ambulatory monitor.

_____

_____

_____ **15.** Emergency equipment should be available in the room or nearby during exercise electrocardiography.

_____

_____

Lead Placement:

16. Draw and label the electrodes for exercise electrocardiography on the figure below.

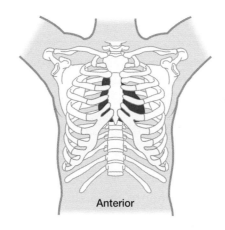

Anterior

Matching

Match these terms with the correct definitions. Place the appropriate letter on the line to the left of each term.

_____ **17.** thallium stress test

_____ **18.** myocardium

_____ **19.** hypertension

_____ **20.** beta blocker

_____ **21.** angiogram

_____ **22.** angina

_____ **23.** dysrhythmia

_____ **24.** cardiologist

_____ **25.** congestive heart failure

_____ **26.** coronary vascular disease

_____ **27.** echocardiogram

_____ **28.** false positive

_____ **29.** THR

a. medication used to treat hypertension

b. pain around the heart caused by lack of oxygen to the heart

c. failure of the heart to pump an adequate amount of blood to the tissue

d. loss of normal rhythm of the heart beat

e. a physician who specializes in the study of the heart

f. x-rays taken of the blood vessels after injection of a radiopaque substance

g. accumulation of plaque and fatty deposits in the coronary arteries

h. noninvasive diagnostic test that uses ultrasound to study the heart and blood vessels

i. when a diagnostic test indicates that disease is present and in reality it is not

j. high blood pressure

k. middle layer of the heart composed of muscle tissue

l. calculated by subtracting your age from 220

m. exercise electrocardiography that is invasive because of injection of a radiopaque substance to view the vessels around the heart

True/False

Read each statement and determine if it is true or false. Circle the T or F. For false (F) statements, correct them to "make them true" on the lines provided.

T   F   **30.** A noninvasive procedure requires entrance into a body cavity, tissue, or blood vessel.

_____

_____

T   F   **31.** A Naughton Protocol is most commonly utilized for a stress test.

_____

_____

T   F   **32.** A Modified Bruce Protocol is most often used during a stress test for patients with an exercise capacity limited by cardiac disease. _____

_____

T   F   **33.** A 12-lead ECG is obtained toward the beginning of each stage of exercise electrocardiography. _____

_____

T   F   **34.** After a stress test, the patient should avoid alcohol, tobacco, and caffeine for at least 3 hours. _____

_____

T   F   **35.** A noninvasive procedure does not require entrance into a body cavity, tissue, or blood vessel. _____

_____

What Should You Do? *Critical Thinking Application*

Read the following situations and use your critical thinking skills to determine how you would handle each. Write your answer in detail in the space provided.

36. Your patient, Mr. Rollins, is scheduled for an exercise electrocardiography test on Friday. When scheduling the appointment, you notice he is taking several heart medications including Atenolol. You check the patient's order and it does not mention whether any of the medications should not be taken before the procedure. Mr. Rollins is getting ready to leave. What should you do?

_____

_____

37. During an exercise electrocardiography procedure, your patient complains of weakness and shortness of breath. He suddenly collapses on the treadmill and falls into the chair. What should you do?

_____

_____

38. Mrs. Annon just had an exercise electrocardiography procedure performed. You are responsible for providing instructions to her before she leaves. After you review the instructions, Mrs. Annon tells you she is going to go for a walk to have a cigarette while she waits for her husband to pick her up. It is about 97° F outside. What should you do?

_____

_____

39. Mr. Wong is required to have a thallium stress test at the outpatient clinic where you are employed. He is a very busy businessman and requests to have the test during his lunch hour. What would be your response?

_____

_____

Get Connected *Internet Activity*

Visit the McGraw-Hill Higher Education Online Learning Center *Electrocardiography for Health Care Personnel* Web site at **www.mhhe.com/healthcareskills** to complete the following activity.

Patient Information for Exercise Electrocardiography Go to the Online Learning Center that accompanies this book and visit the American Heart Association, the National Library of Medicine, and the Heart Health Center Online. Search these and other Web sites to research how frequently exercise electrocardiography is performed and its effectiveness. Be prepared to present your information to the class or prepare your own patient informational brochure.

Using the Student CD

Now that you have completed the material in the chapter text, return to the student CD and complete any chapter activities you have not yet done. Practice your terminology with the "Key Term Concontration" game. Review the chapter material with the "Spin the Wheel" game. Take the final chapter test and complete the troubleshooting question and email or print your results to document your proficiency for this chapter.

7 Ambulatory Monitoring

Learning Outcomes

- Identify the different types of ambulatory monitors and their functions.
- Identify variations of Holter monitoring.
- Explain why ambulatory monitoring is used in addition to the 12-lead ECG.
- List the common uses for ambulatory monitoring.
- Educate the patient about ambulatory monitoring.
- Prepare a patient for application of an ambulatory monitor.
- Apply and remove an ambulatory monitor correctly.
- Identify the procedure for reporting the results from ambulatory monitoring.

Key Terms

ambulate	oscilloscope
anti-arrhythmic	palpitation
dysrhythmia	stress ECG
Holter	syncope

7.1 Introduction

Ambulatory monitoring is the process of recording an ECG tracing for an extended period of time while a patient goes about his or her daily activities, including walking or **ambulating.** A typical ambulatory monitor is a small box that is strapped to the patient's waist or shoulder to record an ECG over a 24- to 48-hour period (see Figure 7-1). Inside the box is a recording device; the entire device usually weighs less than 2 pounds. The most common type looks like a small tape recorder. Newer ambulatory monitors on the market are digital recorders, as seen in Figure 7-2. One type of ambulatory monitor is also known as a **Holter** monitor, named after its inventor, Norman Holter.

Checkpoint Question 7-1

1. How long does a typical ambulatory monitor record an ECG?

_____

_____

Figure 7-1   An ambulatory monitor is attached to the shoulder or waist so the patient is free to move about during the 24- to 48-hour period while the electrical activity of the heart is being recorded.

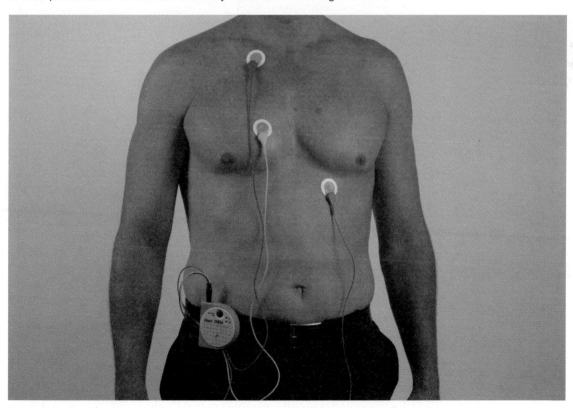

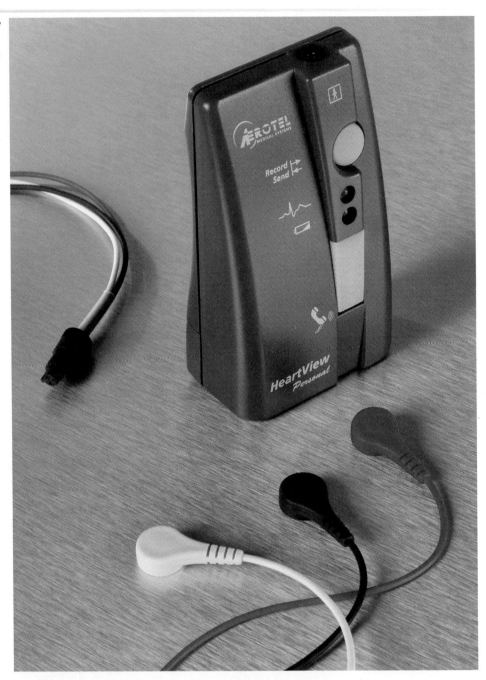

Figure 7-2 Digital ambulatory monitors record the electrical activity of the heart, which can be transferred directly to a computer or over the Internet for interpretation.

7.2 What Is Ambulatory Monitoring?

During ambulatory monitoring, the patient has three to five leads attached to his or her chest, depending on the type of monitor used. The patient may move around and is encouraged to maintain his or her normal daily activities. While the monitor is in place and recording, the patient is asked to keep a diary to record all usual and unusual activities. Any symptoms or abnormal sensations such as chest pain, indigestion, or dizziness should be recorded. If symptoms do occur, the patient is asked to monitor the symptoms and what he or she was doing prior to and during the symptoms. When the monitoring is completed, the information from the monitor and diary must be interpreted. A computer is used to print and/or view the ECG tracing from the monitor. A computer may be used for analysis of the tracing. This computer analysis may be done within the facility, or the tracing may be sent to an outside laboratory, known as a reference laboratory. A physician, usually a cardiologist, does final interpretation of the results. If the results are sent to a reference laboratory, they are returned to the patient's physician.

As a multiskilled health care provider, you will be responsible for applying and removing the ambulatory monitor, providing patient education, and ensuring that the results are placed in the patient's chart. Depending on your place of employment, you may be responsible for scanning the tape or digital disk. The scanner will analyze the data, highlighting any irregularities, or provide a printout for the physician to interpret. Part of your job may be to assist with distinguishing artifact from cardiac dysrhythmias.

Checkpoint Question 7-2

1. What responsibilities might you have for ambulatory monitoring?

   _____

   _____

 Answer the preceding question and complete the "What Is Ambulatory Monitoring?" activity on the student CD under Chapter 7 before you proceed to the next section.

7.3 How Is Ambulatory Monitoring Used?

The purpose of ambulatory monitoring is to document the electrical activity in the heart and identify any abnormal heart behaviors such as dysrhythmias. Abnormal heart behaviors can occur randomly or spontaneously and may be sleep related, disease related, or diet or stress induced. As you have learned in previous chapters, abnormal electrical behavior of the heart can be life threatening.

An ambulatory monitor is used to capture abnormal heart rhythms and correlate symptoms experienced by the patient. For example, a typical patient may be experiencing chest pain, lightheadedness, **syncope** (fainting spells), dizziness, or **palpitations** (rapid, irregular heartbeat). To find the cause of these symptoms, the patient may have already had a 12-lead ECG and a cardiac **stress ECG** (exercise electrocardiography). However, the patient may not have experienced symptoms during these tests, so no abnormal rhythms would have been detected. If the patient is still having symptoms, an ambulatory monitor can be used. During the 24 to 48 hours that the monitor is in place, the patient records all daily activities, abnormal experiences, and symptoms in a diary. The ambulatory monitor provides an ECG tracing at the exact time the patient experiences any symptoms. The physician can interpret the results and evaluate the patient's symptoms based on the ECG tracing.

Ambulatory monitoring is used for other reasons as well. The physician may want to evaluate the effectiveness of cardiac medications such as **anti-arrhythmic** drug therapy (medication given to prevent cardiac rhythm abnormalities). Ambulatory monitoring is also used to evaluate artificial pacemaker functioning. Pacemaker functioning is evaluated after implantation or if problems arise. Ambulatory monitoring can also evaluate the function of the heart after a recent myocardial infarction.

As you can see, ambulatory monitoring is an effective tool to evaluate a wide variety of conditions and problems. However, the decision to use long-term ambulatory monitoring does not come without problems. Education of the patient is essential as discussed throughout this chapter. The patient must have the ability to understand the process. For example, a patient with dementia would not be a good candidate for long-term ambulatory monitoring. Also, the equipment may fail such as with a lead failure wherein the lead quits working during the monitoring process.

Checkpoint Question 7-3

1. Why is a diary a necessary part of Holter monitoring?

_____

_____

 Answer the preceding question and complete the "How Is Ambulatory Monitoring Used?" activity on the student CD under Chapter 7 before you proceed to the next section.

7.4 Functions and Variations

The two most common types of ambulatory monitoring are continuous and intermittent. Continuous monitoring provides a complete tracing of the ECG from the time the monitor is applied until it is removed. During continuous monitoring, the patient may be asked to press a button on the machine to mark the tracing whenever a symptom is felt. This is known as an "event marker." The marker marks the tracing at the exact time the event occurs. The monitor has an accurate clock that indicates the time the marker is applied. The clock is necessary for the physician to be able to correlate the diary entries with what is happening on the ECG tracing.

Intermittent recording records only while the patient is experiencing symptoms. The patient is instructed to press a button on the machine when symptoms occur to start the ECG tracing. The results from this type of tracing are shorter and can be evaluated more quickly than continuous monitoring. However, intermittent monitoring only shows the ECG tracing during the symptoms. Some abnormal rhythms can occur prior to symptoms, and an intermittent recording may not show these abnormalities.

Some ambulatory monitors can be voice activated. When the patient experiences an unusual symptom or changes in activity, he or she can speak into the recorder to describe each event. The event is timed for comparison to the ECG tracing during continuous monitoring. During intermittent monitoring, the ECG tracing may also be activated by the voice. (It is your responsibility to know the type and features of the monitor used in order to properly apply and remove the monitor and instruct the patient.)

Two other variations of ambulatory monitoring include telemetry and transtelephonic monitoring. Telemetry monitoring is performed within a medical facility such as a hospital, whereas transtelephonic monitoring is performed outside the medical facility. Both of these types of monitoring are performed on patients who can ambulate.

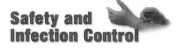
Handle Monitors Carefully

Ambulatory monitors are sensitive and can be very expensive. Be careful when handling an ambulatory monitor. Dropping or hitting the machine against something could cause permanent damage.

Telemetry monitoring is done with a small transmitting device attached to the chest with three or five electrodes (see Figure 7-3). A continuous tracing of the heart is recorded and sent directly to a monitoring station. Telemetry monitors are only transmitting devices designed to send the electrical signal of the heart to a central location to be evaluated continuously. At this location, single or multiple patients may be monitored at the same time on multiple screens (see Figure 7-4). There is no need for a patient diary since the patient is admitted to the facility and will be observed and monitored at all times. In a cardiac intensive care unit, your role as a multiskilled health care giver may include observing the ECG tracings for abnormalities on a

Figure 7-3 At an in-patient facility, patients wear the telemetry monitor leads and the unit attached to the chest. The unit can be placed in the pocket of their gown or on their waist. This allows patients to ambulate and perform activities of daily living during their hospitalization.

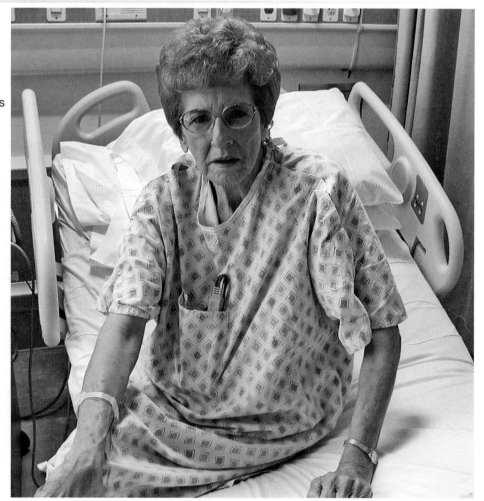

Figure 7-4 Several patients can be monitored simultaneously at a central patient care station. In this picture of an "EICU", the patients being monitored are in another building.

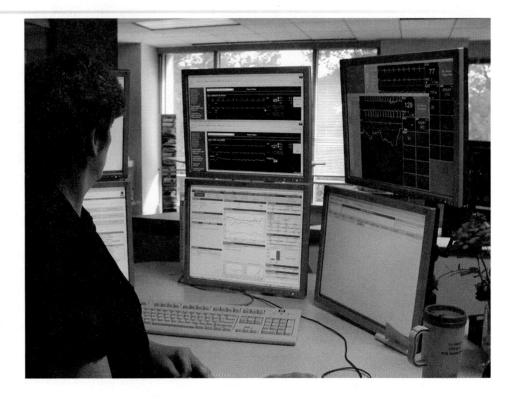

computer-type screen (see Figure 7-5). You will need to be familiar with the **dysrhythmias** (irregularities in heartbeat) presented in Chapter 5. In addition, you may also be required to pass a certification examination to work as a telemetry monitoring technician.

Transtelephonic monitoring was developed in the 1960s after Holter monitoring was developed. It is used mainly to evaluate pacemaker function but is also used for any patient requiring monitoring for longer than 24 to 48

Figure 7-5 Multiple patients can be monitored on a single LCD display screen.

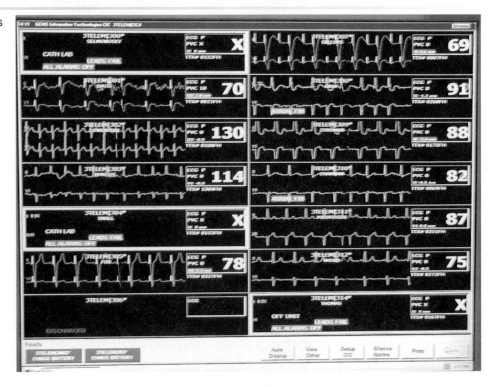

Figure 7-6 Transtelephonic monitors allow information to be transmitted over a phone line or even a cell phone.

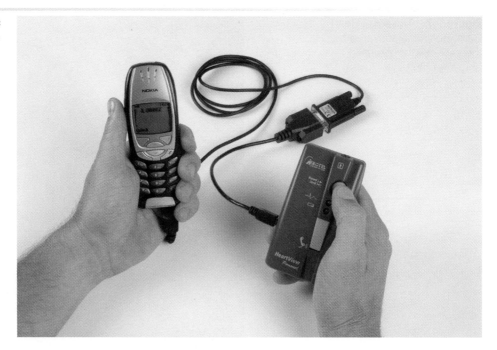

hours. Patients with permanent pacemakers or certain cardiac dysrhythmias may require monitoring for 30 days or more. Transtelephonic monitors are small and portable. The information recorded is stored in the monitor and later transmitted over the telephone line (see Figure 7-6, *A* and *B*).

There are two types of transtelephonic monitors. One type is known as a postsymptom event monitor. This type is used when a patient is experiencing symptoms. It is worn like a wristwatch or it can be handheld. The handheld type should be kept in a convenient place by the patient and is activated when pressed onto the chest (see Figure 7-7). The patient should activate the monitor while experiencing symptoms. The electrode feet on the handheld monitor record a lead II tracing. The wristwatch type is worn at all times and records a two-directional or bipolar lead I tracing. Postsymptom event monitoring records the heart activity for short periods immediately after the patient experiences symptoms. It is used primarily to document dysrhythmias that last more than a few seconds, such as atrial fibrillation, atrial flutter, and supraventricular tachycardias.

Another type of transtelephonic monitor is a loop-memory monitor. This small device is attached to the chest with two lead wires. It remains in place continuously throughout the monitoring period, which may be 30 days or more. The memory on this monitor can hold up to 5 minutes of the ECG tracing and is programmed based on the patient's symptoms and complaints. For example, if a patient has a history of syncope (fainting spells), activating the monitor after an episode will lock the previous 5 minutes of ECG tracing into the memory for transmission over the telephone and evaluation. This provides the physician with an ECG tracing of the heart before, during, and after the episode and helps the physician determine the cause of the syncope (Figure 7-8).

A new "transtelephonic" capability is a 12-lead ECG. This 10-cable device is attached in the same manner and locations discussed in Chapter 4. The difference is that the patient can activate this device any place at any time and send the data to the doctor's office or monitoring facility for

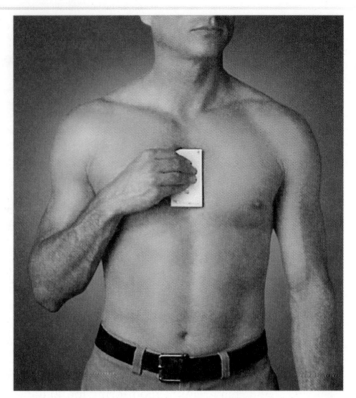

Figure 7-7 The small Heart Card monitor is activated by the patient when pressed onto the chest.

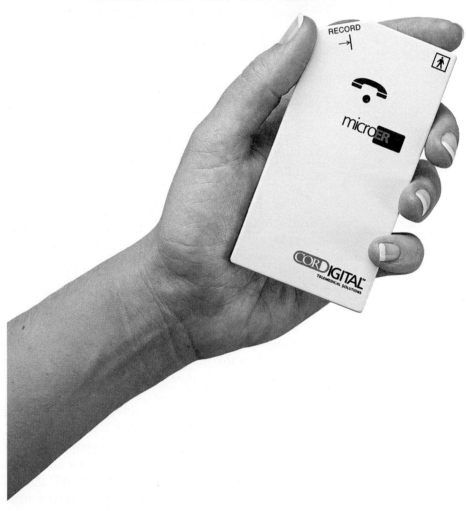

Figure 7-8 The patient presses a button once symptoms begin in order to record all pre- and post-ECG segments.

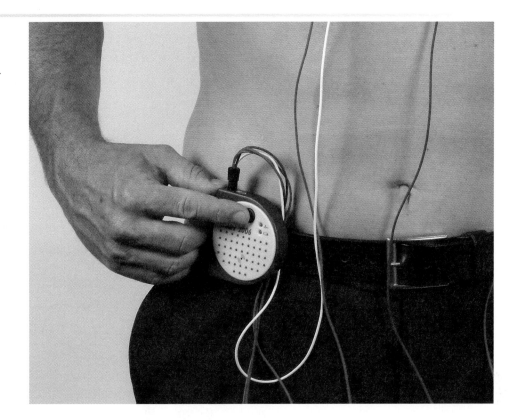

immediate interpretation. This transtelephonic device measures approximately 2½ by 5 inches and weighs only 6 ounces! (See Figure 7-9.)

Troubleshooting **Patient Problems**

Sometimes during ambulatory monitoring the electrodes may become loose or disconnected and the patient will need to know how to handle this situation. Check the policy of the facility where you are employed to give the patient correct instructions. Usually patients are instructed to press loose electrodes in the center to reapply. However, if the electrode comes off completely, the patient will need to report this and return to the facility for replacement. Information about how and when to contact your place of employment should be provided to the patient.

A patient asks you what he should do if an electrode becomes loose. What should you do?

_____

_____

Checkpoint Question 7-4

1. Why is a diary not necessary for telemetry patients?

_____

_____

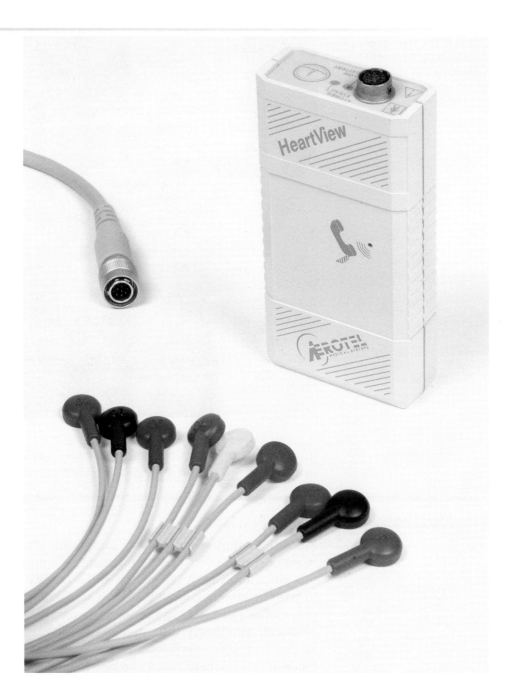

Figure 7-9 Twelve-lead transtelephonic monitor. A 12-lead ECG is produced with this 10-cable transtelephonic monitor.

 Answer the preceding question and complete the "Functions and Variations" activity on the student CD under Chapter 7 before you proceed to the next section.

7.5 Educating the Patient

Prior to having an ambulatory monitor, the patient must be thoroughly instructed on its proper use. Maintaining a diary is vital for accurate interpretation and evaluation of the results of the ECG tracing. The ECG tracing alone is not helpful unless the physician can correlate the results with the activities and symptoms the patient was experiencing during the tracing. Your responsibility is to ensure that the patient understands the monitoring procedure, why it is being done, and what he or she must do while the monitor is in place.

Ensuring Patient Understanding

Begin by asking the patient to tell you what he or she already knows about the ambulatory monitoring procedure. Based on their response, you can then explain to them what they do not know or understand. This is an effective way to ensure that your patient understands the procedure. You should also have the patient repeat the information back to you to demonstrate his or her understanding.

The Patient Diary

The patient diary must be an accurate record of the events and symptoms that occur while the monitor is in place (see Figure 7-10). Most diaries provide time blocks to mark when activities and symptoms occur, making entry easy for the patient (see Figure 7-11). The patient must record *all* activities, including physical and emotional stress and all usual and unusual daily events, such as urinating, bowel movements, sexual activities, walking, emotional upset, eating, and sleeping. You should emphasize the need for an accurate and complete diary. Make sure the patient knows not to change diet or daily activity during ambulatory monitoring.

To ensure that the patient understands the diary recording procedure, have him or her repeat your instructions back to you. You may want the patient to demonstrate his or her understanding by placing a sample entry into the diary. Provide the patient with a complete set of instructions with your name and the facility phone number in the event the patient has any questions or problems. If the patient does not understand how to maintain the diary correctly, the monitoring procedure may have to be repeated. This unnecessary time and expense can be avoided by properly instructing the patient.

Figure 7-10 Explain the importance of the patient diary and the need for an accurate account of the patient's activities during the monitoring. Make sure the patient understands the diary's importance before he or she leaves with an ambulatory monitor.

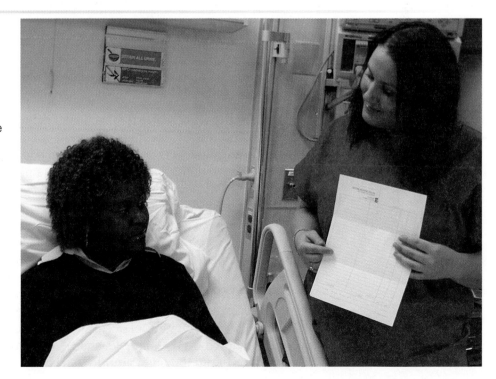

Figure 7-11 Note the sample entries in this Holter monitoring patient diary. The patient should make entries into the diary frequently throughout the Holter monitoring period.

Sample Diary

A portion of a sample diary is shown below. Remember that the more complete your diary, the more value it is for your doctor. If in doubt, write it down. Please print clearly so that your doctor or technician will understand your comments.

TIME	ACTIVITY	SYMPTOM
11:30 am	walking in hall	dizzy
1:45 pm	BM	
2:30 pm	exercise class began	
3:45 pm	sitting watching TV	flutter
11:30	Bed	

Patient Instructions

Carry this diary and a pencil with you at all times and enter your activities, symptoms, and times they occur. Generally you should record:

Time of Day: For every entry in the diary.

Activities: Routine & strenuous exercise, bowel movements, taking medication, or emotional upsets, such as anger.

Symptoms: Chest, neck, arm or face pain, heart pounding, dizziness, nausea, shortness of breath or any other-whether or not you feel they are important. If in doubt, write it down.

Important:
1. Do not tamper with the recorder, electrodes, or electrode leads.
2. Do not get the recorder wet.
3. Your recorder is equipped with a digital clock display and an event marker button; activate it when symptoms occur.

Patient Activity Diary

( )hr   ( )12 hr   ( )24 hr

Patient's Name_____
Patient's Addr._____
_____

Age:_____ Sex:_____
Phone:_____
Medication:_____
_____

Hospital:_____
Room:_____
Date of Recording:_____
Started:_____am/pm
Connected by:_____
_____

As previously mentioned, ambulatory (Holter) monitoring may be done to evaluate the effectiveness of new cardiac medications or the patient's response to discontinuation of cardiac medications. In these circumstances, the physician may change the patient's heart medications prior to the monitoring, either adding a new medication or discontinuing one the patient is currently taking. It is your responsibility to remind the patient of medication changes prescribed by the physician.

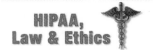

HIPAA, Law & Ethics

Scope of Practice

Licensed practitioners are responsible for educating the patient regarding actions, indications, side effects, and precautions of medications. When a question arises regarding this information, refer the patient to a licensed practitioner to avoid practicing outside the scope of your education and training.

It is best that the patient wear loose fitting clothing during the monitoring procedure for comfort and convenience and to reduce artifact. A front-buttoning shirt is preferred because you can conveniently access the patient's chest and apply the electrodes. The patient must not tamper with the monitor or disconnect the lead wires or electrodes. While the monitor is in place, he or she may take only a sponge bath; no shower or tub bath is allowed during the monitoring because the equipment must not get wet. Patients may sleep in any position that does not apply tension on the lead wires or electrodes. Avoiding magnets, metal detectors, high-voltage areas, and electric blankets is necessary because these devices can interfere with the tracing. The patient should also know how the monitoring equipment works and be instructed to check that it is working properly during the procedure. Documentation of accurate patient education is necessary and must be included on the patient's chart. You may use a paper or electronic checklist similar to the one found in Table 7-1.

TABLE 7-1 Ambulatory Monitoring Checklist

A checklist such as this provides documentation for the medical record of patient instructions for the ambulatory monitoring procedure.

Ambulatory Monitoring—Checklist for Patient Education

Patient Name		
Patient was able to	**YES**	**NO**
• Describe ambulatory monitoring.		
• Explain why he or she is having the test performed.		
• Know the length of time the monitor will be on and when to return the monitor and diary.		
• State where the leads are placed and what they will feel like.		
• Adjust the shoulder strap or waist belt.		
• Wear loose fitting clothing for comfort and convenience.		
• Operate the event marker.		
• Replace loose electrodes and report loose or removed electrodes.		
• Avoid metal detectors, electric detectors, high-voltage wires, and magnets.		
• State required physical restrictions such as bathing, swimming and daily activities.		
• Log usual and unusual activities and symptoms experienced.		
• Contact the facility when necessary.		
Signature	**Date**	**Initials**

Troubleshooting **Patient Instructions**

When reviewing the instructions for the diary with your patient, he asks you if he is allowed to do certain things during the monitoring such as sleep on his stomach or dance at an upcoming dinner party. You should inform him that he is encouraged to participate in his normal daily activities during the monitoring, whatever they may be. Since there is a chance that some activities may cause the electrodes to become loose or disconnected, you should check to be sure he knows the procedure for correcting this situation. You should also explain that if the electrodes become loose or disconnected, it could interfere with the accuracy of the results.

Your patient wants to know if he can continue his daily bike ride while being monitored. What should you say?

_____

_____

**Checkpoint
Question
7-5**

1. Why should the patient wear loose fitting clothing during ambulatory monitoring?

_____

_____

Answer the preceding question and complete the "Educating the Patient" activity on the student CD under Chapter 7 before you proceed to the next section.

7.6 Preparing the Patient

Patients must be prepared for the ambulatory monitoring procedure both emotionally and physically. Many times the patient will be apprehensive. Children may be especially fearful. The first step in reducing the fear is to help them understand the procedure. Take time with the patient to explain each step of the procedure as you perform it. For children, be sure to explain in terms they can understand. Let the patient know it is normal to have some fear and allow the patient to express his or her feelings. Allow the patient to ask questions, and answer as completely as you can. If you do not know the answer, ask a licensed practitioner or your supervisor.

The patient should understand the physical requirements of the monitoring procedure. If the patient is male, he may have to have his chest shaved in order to place the electrodes. For both males and females, there may be some discomfort while the electrodes are in place. You should remind patients that during the procedure they should maintain all regular physical activities.

Patient Education & Communication

Pediatric Patients

Pediatric patients require special consideration when explaining the ambulatory monitoring procedure. Consider the child's age and use terms that he or she will understand. To decrease the child's potential anxieties and fears, allow the patient to touch the equipment prior to applying it. Be sure to instruct the parent as well.

**Checkpoint
Question
7-6**

1. While answering questions for a patient, she asks something and you do not know the answer. What would you say?

_____

_____

Answer the preceding question and complete the "Preparing the Patient" activity on the student CD under Chapter 7 before you proceed to the next section.

7.7 Applying an Ambulatory Monitor

Before the Procedure

Prepare for the procedure by gathering the necessary equipment (see Figure 7-12). You will need the following:

- Monitor with holder and shoulder strap or belt
- New batteries and new tape or disk
- Electrodes (three to five, depending on the type of monitor used)
- Lead wires
- Alcohol and gauze
- Patient diary
- Skin preparation materials (prep pads, benzoin, abrasive cleaner, or skin rasp)
- Shaving equipment
- Tape
- Checklist for patient education
- Manufacturer's directions for specific monitor used
- Pen

Before entering the room to begin the procedure, you should prepare the monitor and review the manufacturer's instructions for the type of monitor you are using. Check to see that the monitor is adequately charged. You will need to insert new batteries to ensure that the monitor will not lose charge during the procedure. Insert a new blank tape or disk if required.

Figure 7-12 Gather all the necessary equipment prior to applying the ambulatory monitor.

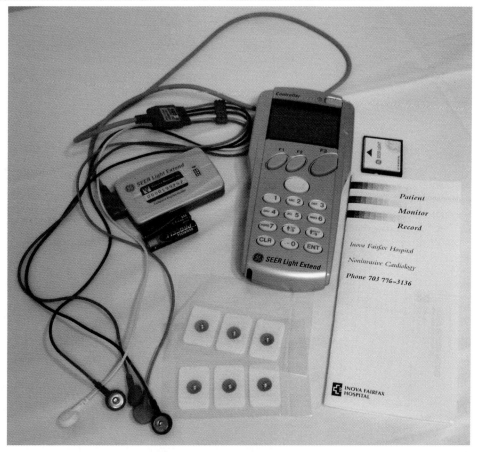

Placing the Electrodes

Have the patient remove his or her clothing from the waist up so you can position the electrodes. You should provide a drape, especially for female patients. Have the patient sit or lie down in a comfortable position on the bed or examination table. The patient should be relaxed.

Prepare the sites for electrode placement. Rub the site with an alcohol swab and let it dry. If the sites are hairy, dry shave the skin. wet shaving is not done because soap film will interfere with electrode adhesion. Use the adhesive side of tape to remove any shaved hair remaining. Abrade the skin using a special prep pad, a dry 4 × 4 gauze, a skin rasp, or another type of abrasive cleaner. Abrading the skin consists of rubbing firmly and briskly at each of the sites where the electrodes will be placed so they will adhere to the skin better. Preparation of the electrode sites may vary depending on the type of ambulatory monitoring performed. For telemetry monitoring, it is recommended that the chest hair be *clipped* and not shaved. This prevents irritation and keeps the patient from scratching, which can cause artifact on the tracing. Check the manufacturer's instructions and the policy of your facility for proper electrode placement.

Safety and Infection Control

Elderly Patients

Elderly patients and patients taking certain medications may have very fragile, thin skin. Manipulate the electrodes as little as possible when applying and removing them, and use care to prevent skin damage or pain. You should apply less pressure when abrading the skin and avoid abrasive cleaners when preparing the sites.

Place the electrodes on the chest at the proper sites. See Figure 7-13 for one example. Electrode placement depends on the number of lead wires, the type of monitor used, and the lead tracing to be produced. Check the manufacturer's instructions for accurate placement of the electrodes for the monitor you are using. If the leadwires are the "snap-on" type, you should

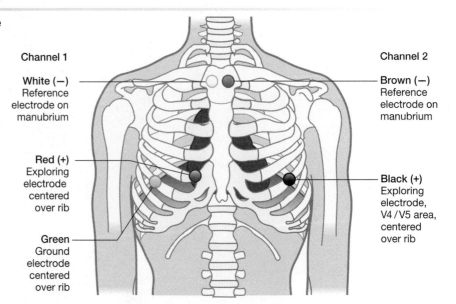

Figure 7-13 This is one example of 5-lead electrode placement for ambulatory monitoring. Lead placement may vary, so check the manufacturer's instructions for the correct placement for the monitor you wil be using.

Channel 1

White (−)
Reference electrode on manubrium

Red (+)
Exploring electrode centered over rib

Green
Ground electrode centered over rib

Channel 2

Brown (−)
Reference electrode on manubrium

Black (+)
Exploring electrode, V4/V5 area, centered over rib

attach the electrodes to the lead wires prior to placing them on the patient to reduce discomfort. Remove the backing from the adhesive, then apply each electrode to its proper position by pressing firmly at the center. Run your finger around the edge of each electrode to ensure firm attachment.

Attach the lead wires to the electrodes. Check the wire color and cable identification to ensure proper attachment to the electrode. Arrange the lead wires and cable comfortably on the patient. Tape each of the electrodes in place to reduce tugging and pulling on the electrodes during movement. Some electrodes include stress loops to reduce artifact. (See Figure 7-14)

Attach the cable to an electrocardiograph and run a baseline ECG tracing. Make sure the tracing is correct and that the machine is not malfunctioning. Have the patient put on his or her shirt and run the lead wire between the buttons or out the bottom of the shirt. Attach the cable to the monitor, place it in the carrying case, and attach it comfortably to the patient's waist or shoulder. Double-check the lead wires and electrodes to ensure that there is no pulling on them.

Start the monitor and have the patient place the first entry into the diary. Make sure the beginning time is noted in the diary. Review all instructions with the patient and set the date and time for him or her to return for removal. Make sure the patient knows how to get assistance in case problems arise.

Checkpoint Question 7-7

1. What kind of problems could the patient encounter during monitoring?

_____

_____

Answer the preceding question and complete the "Applying an Ambulatory Monitor" activity on the student CD under Chapter 7 before you proceed to the next section.

Figure 7-14 Individual stress loops take up slack and prevent tension on the lead wires and electrodes during ambulatory monitoring.

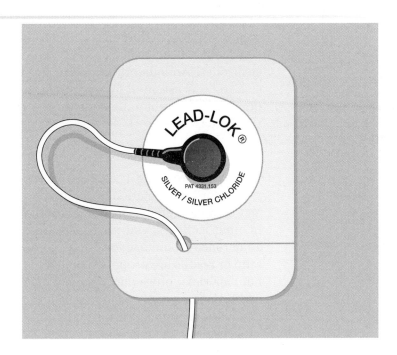

7.8 Removing an Ambulatory Monitor and Reporting Results

When the patient returns to have the monitor removed, briefly review the completed diary with him or her. Turn off the monitor and detach it from the lead wires, then detach the lead wires and cables from the patient. Remove the tape and electrodes from the patient's chest. Clean the skin where the electrodes had been placed. Record the removal procedure on the patient's chart.

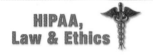

HIPAA, Law & Ethics

Document and Label

Carefully document and label the report, diary, and tape or digital disk with all required information as established by the facility protocol.

Once the monitoring is complete, your next responsibility is to see that the results are evaluated and a report is placed in the medical record. In order for the results of the recording to be evaluated, they must be put in the proper format. Each type and brand of ambulatory monitor has a slightly different procedure for preparing the recording for analysis. In some circumstances, you may need to attach the machine to a scanner or computer. The recording will be viewed on an output device such as a monitor, **oscilloscope,** or printer. The computer may provide an analysis as well. A physician, usually a cardiologist, must view the recording and the patient diary in order for a final interpretation to be completed. Computer interpretation and evaluation by a cardiologist may occur within your facility, or the monitor cassette may be sent to an outside laboratory, known as a reference laboratory, for analysis.

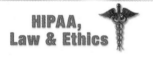

HIPAA, Law & Ethics

Ensure Accurate Results

You are assigned to apply a new type of Holter monitor that has a five-lead system. Since you have never used this type of five-lead system before, you should first check the manufacturer's instructions prior to placing the electrodes. Ambulatory monitors can vary, and correct placement of the electrodes is essential for accurate results. If you cannot locate the directions or still do not understand the correct placement, you should consult your supervisor.

If you are using a cassette-recorder-type monitor, you will need to prepare it for interpretation. This involves preparing the ECG tracing printout and computer analysis, along with the diary, for the physician to interpret. In other facilities, you may only have to remove the cassette and send it to a reference laboratory for interpretation. In either case, make sure the cassette or results are properly labeled with the patient's name, medical record number, date, physician's name, and any other identifying information. In addition, the patient's diary must be kept with the cassette or printed results. Check the manufacturer's information provided with the monitor and your supervisor for specific instructions.

Accurate results must be provided for correct interpretation of the ECG tracing. Many factors can affect these results such as improper lead attachment, incomplete patient diary, and failure of the patient to maintain a normal routine. You can reduce the chances of having to repeat the procedure by ensuring proper lead attachment, patient education, and recording of results. The test may need to be repeated if the results are inconclusive.

When the results are sent to an outside lab, it usually takes 7 to 10 days to get the report. The final report must be placed on the patient's chart for the physician to provide the patient with the results of the test. Abnormal results may indicate any of the following:

- Electrical-conduction defects in the heart's rate and rhythm-controlling system
- Rhythm abnormalities
- Premature atrial or ventricular contractions

Troubleshooting **No Diary**

When your patient returns to have his or her monitor removed, you should first ask for the patient diary. If the patient has forgotten to bring the diary, the results of the recording cannot be evaluated.

What do you think you should do if a patient arrives without the diary?

_____

_____

Advise your patient to discuss the results of the ambulatory monitoring with his or her physician. It is important to note that the ambulatory monitor is only part of the diagnostic process. Results of the Holter monitoring will correlate the patient's symptoms with changes on the ECG tracing. Additional tests may be required, depending on the patient's condition. Some examples include the following:

- Echocardiogram
- Coronary angiogram
- CT (computerized tomography) scan
- MRI (magnetic resonance imaging) scan
- PET (positron emission tomography) scan

Checkpoint Question 7-8

1. What factors can affect the results of ambulatory monitoring?

_____

_____

 Answer the preceding question and complete the "Removing an Ambulatory Monitor and Reporting Results" activity on the student CD under Chapter 7.

Chapter Summary

- The most common type of ambulatory monitor is the Holter monitor. Telemetry for inpatients and transtelephonic for outpatients monitoring are also common.

- Ambulatory monitoring can be either continuous or intermittent. Intermittent only records when the patient is experiencing symptoms and the tracing is shorter. During continuous monitoring the patient uses an event marker or voice activation.

- Unlike an ECG which evaluates the heart at one point in time, ambulatory monitoring is used to evaluate the ECG during a long period of time when symptoms or problems could occur.

- Ambulatory monitoring is used to evaluate for dysrhythmias and correlate them to symptoms the patient is experiencing, to evaluate the effectiveness of cardiac medications, and to check the functioning of an artificial pacemaker.

- The patient undergoing ambulatory monitoring must be educated about the procedure, its reasons, how long and when to return, the equipment including marking the tracing during symptoms and electrode problems, the diary, and when and how to contact the medical facility.

- After educating the patient, the equipment must be gathered and prepared, and the electrodes are placed on the patient's chest.

- Before removing the monitor the diary must be completed by the patient, then turn off the recording, remove the leads, clean the skin, and report the results.

- The recording must be prepared for review and evaluation. This process is based upon the type of equipment used.

Chapter Review

Ordering:

The following is a list of steps for applying the ambulatory monitor. Number the steps in sequential order from 1 to 13.

_____ **1.** Prepare the chest for lead placement.

_____ **2.** Identify the patient.

_____ **3.** Remove the patient's clothes from the waist up and use a drape for female patients.

_____ **4.** Explain the procedure.

_____ **5.** Record the procedure in the patient's chart.

_____ **6.** Attach the lead wires.

_____ **7.** Record the start time in the patient's diary.

_____ **8.** Start the monitor and make sure that it is functioning correctly.

_____ **9.** Remove the adhesive backing and apply the electrodes at the correct sites.

_____ **10.** Place the monitor in its holder and strap it comfortably to the patient.

_____ **11.** Give the patient the diary and review the instructions.

_____ **12.** Attach the cable to the monitor.

_____ **13.** Secure the lead wires to the electrodes with tape.

Matching:

Match the key terms with their definitions. Place the correct letter on the line provided.

_____ **14.** Holter

_____ **15.** palpitation

_____ **16.** stress ECG

_____ **17.** myocardial infarction

_____ **18.** syncope

_____ **19.** oscilloscope

_____ **20.** dysrhythmia

_____ **21.** ambulate

_____ **22.** anti-arrhythmic

a. walk

b. medication given to prevent arrhythmias

c. irregularity or loss of rhythm of the heartbeat

d. ambulatory monitor

e. heart attack

f. monitor or TV-type device used to view the ECG

g. fast, irregular heartbeat sensation felt by the patient

h. exercise electrocardiography

i. fainting

Patient Education:

You are assigned to teach Mr. Booth about ambulatory monitoring. From the following list, determine which are correct patient instructions for ambulatory monitoring and which are not. Place a *C* beside the correct statements and an *I* beside the incorrect statements. For each of the incorrect (*I*) statements, write the correct instructions for the patient.

_____ 23. You should avoid alcohol and caffeine during ambulatory monitoring.

_____

_____

_____ 24. During ambulatory monitoring, you will need to record your activities and any symptoms in your diary.

_____

_____

_____ 25. Mr. Booth, you may take a tub bath as long as you do not let the monitor drop into the water.

_____

_____

_____ 26. Wear a loose fitting shirt, preferably one that buttons down the front, and you will be more comfortable during the procedure.

_____

_____

_____ 27. Mr. Booth, you should not take your heart medications during the ambulatory monitoring procedure unless instructed to do so by the physician.

_____

_____

Multiple Choice:

Circle the correct answer for each of the following.

28. Mr. Jones will be attached to a transtelephonic monitor. How long will he have the monitor in place?
    a. 2 to 4 hours
    b. 24 to 48 hours
    c. Up to 30 days
    d. Only during his hospital stay

29. Ms. Buckwalter is attached to a telemetry monitor. How long will she have the monitor in place?
    a. 2 to 4 hours
    b. 24 to 48 hours
    c. Up to 30 days
    d. Only during her hospital stay

30. Mr. Casler is having an ambulatory (Holter) monitor attached and asks you how long it will remain in place. Your answer would be
    a. "2 to 4 hours."
    b. "24 to 48 hours."
    c. "Up to 30 days."
    d. "Only during his hospital stay."

31. Your patient Mrs. Jackson asks, "Why am I having this ambulatory monitor attached when I just had an ECG the other day?" What would be your *best* answer?
    a. "Ambulatory monitors record your heart activity in a different way than an ECG does."
    b. "Your doctor wants to find out what is happening to your heart during a longer period of time than an ECG."
    c. "It is necessary to monitor your heart while you are walking. That is why it is called ambulatory monitoring."
    d. "I cannot answer that question. You should speak to your doctor."

32. Which of the following is *not* a common use of the ambulatory monitor?
    a. To monitor the heart during exercise
    b. To monitor the heart during a typical day
    c. To evaluate pacemaker function
    d. To correlate symptoms and heart activity

Lead Placement:

Label the color and placement of the electrodes on the lines provided.

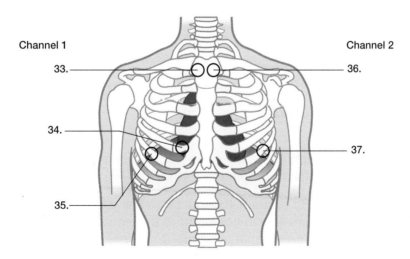

Channel 1   Channel 2

33. _____

34. _____

35. _____

36. _____

37. _____

What Should You Do? *Critical Thinking Application*

Read the following situations and use critical thinking skills to determine how you would handle each. Write your answer in detail in the space provided.

38. While working in an ambulatory care facility, you are preparing an ambulatory monitor for placement. You are about to insert the batteries when the monitor slips out of your hands. You are by yourself and no one sees or hears you drop the monitor. What should you do?

_____

_____

39. When a patient returns to have his or her monitor removed, you check the patient's diary. You notice that many places have been left blank and the diary does not appear complete. What should you do?

_____

_____

40. Mr. Hernandez, a 67-year-old man with a pacemaker, has just had his monitor applied. You ask Mr. Hernandez to enter the first entry into his diary before he leaves. He appears hesitant. You try to encourage him and he flatly refuses. What should you do?

_____

_____

41. You are applying an ambulatory monitor to Ms. Lin. She states that she will be picking up her brother at the airport tomorrow before she returns to have the monitor removed. Should this be a concern to you or Ms. Lin? How would you respond to her statement? Is there a reason why Ms. Lin should or should not go to the airport, and if so, what is it?

_____

_____

Get Connected *Internet Activity*

Visit the McGraw-Hill Higher Education *Electrocardiography for Health Care Personnel* Web site at the **www.mhhe.com/healthcareskills** to complete the following activity.

Visit the Web MD Internet site and/or perform a search to review patient information about the ambulatory monitoring. Consider how you might simplify the explanation of the ambulatory monitoring procedure to a child. What comparisons could you make? Write a paragraph explaining how you would describe the procedure to a 6-year-old, a 10-year-old, or 2-year-old.

Using the Student CD

Now that you have completed the material in the chapter text, return to the student CD and complete any chapter activities you have not yet done. Practice your terminology with the "Key Term Concentration" game. Review the chapter material with the "Spin the Wheel" game. Take the final chapter test and complete the troubleshooting question and email or print your results to document your proficiency for this chapter.

Appendix A

Competency Checklists

Procedure Checklist 4-1

Recording an Electrocardiogram

Step	Rationale	Performed Yes No	Mastered
Preprocedure			
1. Receive and validate order.			
2. Check machine for proper functioning including electrical cord, lead wires, and paper.			
3. Obtain necessary supplies.			
4. Read specific information from manufacturer's instructions.			
5. Ensure adequate paper.			
6. Change or add paper if necessary.			
7. Enter data into ECG machine if available.			
Procedure			
1. Identify patient using two forms of identification.	• Ensures HIPAA standards		
2. Explain procedure.			
3. Wash hands.			
4. Position and prepare patient. Turn off and remove electronics.	• Prevents artifact		
5. Provide for privacy and prevent exposure.	• Provides comfort, alleviates stress		
6. Ensure bed or exam table is not touching wall.	• Prevents artifact		

(Continued)

Step	Rationale	Performed		Mastered
		Yes	No	
Procedure (*continued*)				
7. Move the bed or exam table away from electrical equipment.	• Prevents artifact			
8. Ensure patient is not touching headboard, footboard, or side rails.	• Prevents artifact			
9. Cleanse and prepare skin as necessary.				
10. Apply electrodes to limbs and chest.				
11. Attach lead wire, assuming that no tension is on wires. Make a stress loop.	• Prevents discomfort to patient and artifact			
12. Enter additional patient data in the LCD panel if necessary.				
13. Press Run button.				
14. Check tracing for quality. Observe for artifact.				
15. Run additional ECG if necessary.				
16. Observe LCD display for errors.				
17. Turn off machine and unplug when completed.				
18. Remove electrodes and clean skin, if necessary.				
19. Assist the patient to a safe and comfortable position.				
Postprocedure				
1. Write on ECG any variations in lead placement, reason for poor quality tracing, or change in tracing speed.	• Ensures accurate evaluation			
2. Provide the results to the licensed practitioner.				
3. Place completed ECG tracing in the appropriate area.				
4. Clean the leads.				
5. Drape the lead wires of the machine in an orderly fashion.				
6. Return the machine to the designated storage location.				

Comments:

_____

_____

_____

_____

_____

Signed

Evaluator: _____

Student: _____

Competency Checklist 6-1

Assisting with Exercise Electrocardiography (Stress Testing)

Procedure Step	Rationale	Performed		Mastered
		Yes	No	
Preprocedure: Setting the Appointment				
1. Verify that the medical history is complete.	• To ensure safety and accurate testing			
2. Explain the procedure including reason for test, possible complications, and all safety measures that will be followed during procedure.				
3. Explain "Informed Consent" and ask patient to sign consent form.				
4. Inform patient that day of test he or she should wear comfortable clothing (shorts or gym suit, tennis shoes). Refrain from use of tobacco, caffeine, or alcohol for AT LEAST 3 HOURS prior to test. Patient should eat a light meal 2 hours prior to test.	• The effects of tobacco, caffeine, or alcohol could affect the results of the test.			
5. Check the physician's order against the patient medication list to provide information as to what medications patient should *not* take day of test.	• Certain medications can affect the results of the test.			
6. Go over all instructions and information with the patient. Encourage questions and ask the patient to repeat important information back to you.	• To make sure patient fully understands procedure			
7. Provide a copy of the detailed list of instructions making sure that facility telephone number and your name appear on list. Encourage patient to call if he or she has any questions prior to test day.				
Procedure: Day of Appointment				
1. Verify that the equipment is in working order and supplies are on hand including plenty of tracing paper. Be certain to inspect the cables; make sure the treadmill and computer are working and the correct protocol is determined.	• To prevent problems during the procedure when the patient and physician are present			
2. Gather all supplies including electrodes, alcohol, gauze sponges, razor, adhesive tape, and blood pressure cuff.				
3. Check that the crash cart is ready and fully supplied with the defibrillator working.				
4. Verify the physician's order, that the medical history is complete, and that the informed consent is signed.				
5. Bring the patient into the room.				

6. Verify with the patient that he or she has complied with all instructions.

7. Provide patient with privacy to change into gown with opening to front. Assist if necessary.
   - Opening needs to be in the front in order to place leads.

8. Assist patient to lie down on table.
   - Provides for safety

9. Prepare the skin and apply electrodes as indicated by protocol of facility or equipment manual.

10. Connect the cables, apply the blood pressure cuff, and check ECG tracing for artifact.
    - Ensures proper results during the examination.

11. Obtain blood pressure and ECG in the following positions. Assist as necessary.
    - Supine
    - Sitting
    - Sitting, post 30-second hyperventilation
    - Standing

    - Provides for safety of patient

12. Change the resting position in stress test machine and enter new blood pressure for each tracing.

13. Demonstrate the treadmill including the proper posture and holding the hand grip.
    - Prevents falls

14. Explain the test protocol, making sure the patient understands that the speed and incline will increase every 3 minutes during test phase.

15. Be sure patient understands that he or she is to report any pain, shortness of breath, faintness, tingling sensations, numbness, or extreme fatigue immediately.
    - Provides for safety of patient

16. Watch the patient closely during the test looking for visual signs of any pain, shortness of breath, faintness, tingling sensations, numbness, or extreme fatigue.
    - Provides for safety of patient

17. Ask patient repeatedly during procedure how he or she feels.
    - Provides for safety of patient

18. Explain to the patient again that the test will be completed when target heart rate (THR) is reached. [THR = (220 − age) × 0.85] or when the patient cannot continue due to fatigue or other symptoms.

19. Inform the physician that the patient is ready to begin test.
    - The physician must be present during the procedure.

20. When the physician is in the room, assist patient to the treadmill, making sure patient's feet are not on the belt.

(Continued)

Procedure Step	Rationale	Performed Yes	No	Mastered

Procedure: Day of Appointment (*continued*)

21. Start the belt, tell patient to get used to speed and then to step onto the belt. Ask patient if he or she is ready to begin, explaining again that belt speed and incline will increase. Begin the test phase.

22. At the two and one-half minute mark of each phase take the blood pressure and enter the data into computer. Remind patient before every transition to new phase and be ready to assist the patient as needed.
- Provides for safety

23. When treadmill phase of test is complete by either the THR reached or the patient cannot continue, assist patient to waiting chair.
- Provides for safety

Postprocedure Posttest

1. Continue to monitor and observe the patient's condition closely, taking the blood pressure, entering the data, and then taking an ECG tracing every 3 to 5 minutes for 10 to 15 minutes.
- Verifies the patient condition and tolerance of the testing procedure

2. After the 10-to-15-minute cooldown period, remove the cables and electrodes and wipe off any remaining gel or adhesive.

3. Allow patient to dress (assist if needed).

4. Explain to patient that he or she should avoid tobacco, caffeine, alcohol for at least 3 hours. Patient should avoid extreme temperature changes, including hot shower or bath for 2 hours. Patient should rest and recuperate after test.
- Provides for safety

5. Explain that the physician will have the results of the test in 10 days. Thank the patient for his or her participation.

6. File the results and report per the protocol of the facility.

7. Make sure all information from patient chart is returned to its proper place.
- Maintains HIPAA

Comments: _____

_____

_____

_____

Signed

Evaluator: _____

Student: _____

Procedure Checklist 7-1

Applying and Removing an Ambulatory (Holter) Monitor

Procedure Step	Rationale	Performed		Mastered
		Yes	No	
Preprocedure				
1. Gather supplies and equipment.				
• Prep razor				
• Alcohol				
• Electrodes				
• Gauze pads				
• Skin rasp				
• Tape				
• Holter unit with strap and case				
• Fresh batteries				
• New cassette tape or digital disk				
• Pen and patient diary				
2. Review patient instructions per facility policy.	• To ensure accuracy and prevent problems during the testing procedure			
• Documentation (diary), activities of daily living (ADLs), when symptoms occur				
• Medications				
• Physical restrictions such as new activities (should maintain normal routine), bathing, showers, swimming while wearing the device				
• How to operate the "event" marker				
• How to reapply electrode if one comes loose or falls off				
• Must return with the Holter and diary to complete the test				
• Must wear loose fitting garments on the upper body to reduce artifact				

(Continued)

Procedure Step	Rationale	Performed		Mastered
		Yes	No	
Preprocedure (*continued*)				
• Provide facility phone number, copy of instructions, and "point of contact" if the patient has questions, problems or concerns.				
• Provide picture of electrode locations, extra electrodes, and adhesive tape per clinic policy.				
Procedure				
1. Electrode application				
• Using alcohol pads, gently rub and cleanse the patient's skin to obtain a good skin-to-electrode contact.	• Reduces artifact			
• Dry each site completely by rubbing the skin with a gauze pad until it is dry.				
• Shave and/or clip any hair in the areas where the electrodes will be attached.				
• Wrap tape with adhesive side facing outward from hand and pat gently to remove any loose hairs remaining on the patient's skin.				
• Remove the electrodes from their package and snap onto the patient leads.	• Prevents pressure on the patient's chest caused by applying leads to electrodes when placed on chest			
• Peel the protective backing off the electrodes one at a time as they are placed on the patient.				
2. Lead placement				
• Place electrodes in the appropriate position. (Follow the physician's preference or manufacturer's instructions.)				
• Try to center the electrodes over the ribs by gently setting the gelled center against the skin.	• A wrinkled electrode or dispersed gel would cause an inaccurate tracing.			
• If the electrode wrinkles or gel is dispersed, apply a new electrode.				
• Form a stress loop for each electrode and tape the cable, loop, and electrode to the skin.				

- Leave enough slack between the electrode and the stress loop to allow the patient to move without pulling or stressing the electrodes.

- Verify that all leads are firmly inserted into the monitor.

- Prevents inaccurate tracing

3. **Prepare equipment**

- Insert the digital flashcard or cassette into the recorder.

- Insert appropriate number and size of new batteries into the recorder.

- Once the batteries have been inserted, DO NOT remove the flashcard; doing so will render the flashcard unusable until it has been reinitialized by a scan technician.

- Slide and secure the battery cover onto the recorder.

- An LED may blink as the recorder performs an initialization sequence and self-diagnostics. This will take approximately 20 seconds.

4. **Starting the recording**

- Wait for the green LED to stop flashing and stay lit. This indicates the recorder is collecting ECG data and functioning properly.

- Note start time on enrollment form and patient's diary.

- Place recorder in pouch and review instructions with the patient.

- Have patient sign the Patient Responsibility Statement on the enrollment form.

- Complete paperwork.

Postprocedure

1. Ending the recording

- Collect the patient diary—check to ensure entries were made.

- Check with the patient to make sure no problems occurred during the recording procedure.

(Continued)

Procedure Step	Rationale	Performed		Mastered
		Yes	No	

Postprocedure (*continued*)

Procedure Step	Rationale	Yes	No	Mastered
• Report problems to the licensed practitioner per facility policy.				
• Turn off and disconnect the device per manufacturer's instructions.				
• Disconnect the cable from the Holter unit.				
• Remove the recorder from the pouch.				
• Carefully remove electrodes from patient.	• Prevents irritation and tearing of the skin, especially for patient with paper-thin skin			
• Clean any residual electrode gel from the patient's skin and assist the patient as necessary.				
• Remove and discard the batteries.				
• Remove the flashcard/tape from the recorder.				
• Remove excess tapes and clean cables with a nonalcohol adhesive remover				
• Turn in recording and diary for analysis per facility policy.				
• Document completed procedure according to your facility policy.				
• Explain to the patient that results may take 7 to 10 days and when he or she will be notified of the results.				

Comments: _____

_____

_____

Signed

Evaluator: _____

Student: _____

Cardiovascular Medications

Beta Blockers

Drugs in this class include:

- Atenol**ol**
- Metoprol**ol**
- Propranol**ol**
- Sotal**ol**
- Labetol**ol**
- Digoxin

Note: The majority of drugs in this class end in *ol*.

Beta blockers are used to treat angina pectoris (chest pain caused by lack of blood/oxygen to the heart muscle), hypertension (high blood pressure, various heart rhythm disturbances such as atrial fibrillation, and PVCs. Digoxin is a well-known drug extracted from the foxglove plant. Digoxin increases the force of the heart's contractions and slows the heart rate as well. This medication is especially helpful in treating patients with congestive heart failure (CHF). Digoxin is specifically a medication with a host of side effects (i.e., visual disturbances, various cardiac dysrhythmias, and even depression of the ST segment).

Calcium Channel Blockers

Calcium channel blockers are used to treat a variety of cardiac conditions including hypertension, angina pectoris, and certain types of rapid heart beat conditions. They are also used to treat coronary artery spasms.

Ace Inhibitors

Drugs in this class include:

- Enalapr**il**
- Lisinopr**il**
- Captopr**il**
- Accupr**il**

Note: The majority of drugs in this class end in *il*.

The angiotensin converting enzyme (ACE) inhibitors are named because they work by inhibiting (blocking) the conversion of angiotensin

I to angiotensin II in the lungs. Angiotensin II is a potent hormone that constricts arterioles and raises blood pressure. As a result, ACE inhibitors lower the blood pressure. ACE inhibitors are also used in the treatment of patients with congestive heart failure. They work by lowering the overall resistance in the vascular beds, making it easier for the heart to pump the blood.

Anti-arrhythmic Medications

The first medication found to be useful in treating disorders of the heartbeat was Digitalis leaf. It has been used for over 100 years to treat atrial fibrillation and congestive heart failure. It is still commonly used in a modified form today. There are many different classes of anti-arrhythmic medications because the electrical conduction system of the heart is so complex. Each anti-arrhythmic-class medication affects the speed or way that electricity flows through the heart.

Blood Thinners

Drugs in this class include:

- Coumadin
- Aspirin
- Plavix
- Heparin
- Lovenox

This group of drugs is extremely useful in the treatment of blood clot conditions. These medications are administered by a number of different methods. Although some may be administered in more than one way, they all are not administered the same way and not for all the same reasons. These medications all work to prevent clots from forming or to prevent existing clots from enlarging. They *do not* lyse (break up or destroy) existing clots.

- **Oral Medications**

    Coumadin (warfarin) is the most commonly prescribed outpatient "blood thinner." It is prescribed in the treatment of heart valve conditions (including patients with artificial valves and for valve prolapse when blood is not flowing in the proper direction). It is also prescribed for other medical conditions in which blood clotting is a problem and embolization is a risk.

    Aspirin is a very potent anticoagulant that has been found to lower the risk of heart attacks as well as improving the prognosis with a heart attack. Data have also shown a reduced stroke risk in patients who take prophylactic aspirin. It is a first-line drug administered to "chest pain" patients presenting for emergency care of acute coronary syndromes. Aspirin is routinely prescribed to men over 40 years and postmenopausal women to reduce their risk of clot formation.

    Plavix (antiplatelet drug) was developed approximately 5 years ago. It is another class of "blood thinners." It is useful in angioplasty/coronary stent implantation to prevent postprocedure closure of the treated artery.

- **Intravenous or Subcutaneous Medications**

  Heparin and **Lovenox** are very potent intravenous blood thinners. This type of thinner is generally used in an inpatient setting to quickly stop the development of an ongoing blood clot as seen in serious unstable angina, certain strokes, and acute pulmonary embolism. They have no effect on blood platelets.

  Warfarin (as previously noted) is primarily used in the treatment of atrial fibrillation and in patients who have artificial metallic heart valves. Warfarin use significantly reduces the risk of embolism development in patients with atrial fibrillation.

Fibrinolytics

Also known as "clot busters," these medications are most commonly used in an inpatient setting where they rapidly dissolve clots wherever they are located (i.e., inside a heart artery causing a heart attack, or inside a brain artery causing a stroke). The clot is lysed quickly once the clot buster is administered. These drugs can also be used to treat large pulmonary embolisms and clots causing obstruction of a prosthetic (metallic) valve.

Because of the way clot busters work, when administered they can increase the risk of bleeding elsewhere in the body (IV site, intracranial, etc.). Unfortunately, the category of people with the greatest need of these medications are also at the greatest risk for complications as a result of this medication.

Diuretics

Diuretics act by removing salt and water from the body through the action of the kidneys (elimination). Diuretics are used primarily in the treatment of congestive heart failure (CHF) and are often used in the treatment of hypertension (high blood pressure). **Caution** must be observed when treating patients with diuretics as salt and water are not the only elements removed by the action of medications in this class. Other essential electrolytes may be eliminated as well (i.e., potassium, calcium, magnesium, etc.), which may contribute to the development of cardiac dysrhythmias.

Cholesterol-Lowering Medicines (Statins)

Cholesterol-lowering medications work to lower the LDL ("bad") cholesterol in the blood. Some of these drugs also raise the HDL ("good") cholesterol. This class of drugs has been shown to reduce the incidence of heart attack and death in patients with high cholesterol and coronary artery disease.

Promising research is being reported that elevated doses of certain statins may actually reverse atherosclerotic plaque within blood vessels, thereby reducing the potential for sudden cardiac death and reducing potentially the need for surgical intervention. There are always drawbacks: This category of medications is also potentially hepatotoxic, and high doses of statins may in some cases destroy the liver.

Nitrates

Nitrates are the most commonly prescribed vasodilators, or medications that widen the blood vessels. They are frequently used for relief of ischemic chest pain in patients with coronary vascular disease and angina (chest pain). They work by relaxing smooth muscles, most notably the muscles of the heart and blood vessels. As a result, pressure on blood vessel walls is reduced, which allows more blood to circulate with less effort by the heart. Nitrates affect veins as well as arteries, but their vasodilatory effect is more pronounced on veins. Nitrates prevent and relieve angina by relieving vasoconstriction and restoring blood flow and oxygen to ischemic heart muscle.

Nitrates can be administered intravenously, sublingually (via metered spray or tablet), transdermally (ointments or skin patches), and orally.

Safety note: Don't ever handle nitrates with your bare hands!

Of Particular Concern to Patients Taking Nitrates

- Any medication that is already being taken to treat hypertension and/or **erectile dysfunction medications** (e.g., Viagra, Cialis, Levitra). When taken in combination, these can increase the effects of nitrates on blood pressure, causing profound irreversible hypotension, cardiac arrest, and even death.

Inotropes (Also Known as Cardiotonics)

Drugs in this class include:

- Adenosine
- Digitalis (Digitoxin, Digoxin)
- Dobutamine.

These medications strengthen the pumping action of the heart and, as a result, reduce cardiac workload (myocardial oxygen demand). They are commonly used to treat patients with heart failure or tachydysrhythmias.

Appendix C

Medical Abbreviations, Acronyms, and Symbols

The following are common medical abbreviations, acronyms, and symbols. Always check the facility where you are employed for the acceptable medical abbreviations, acronyms, and symbols used.

Medical Abbreviation	Term
Numbers	
1°	First degree
2°	Second degree
2de	Two-dimensional echocardiography
3°	Third degree
A	
a k amputation	Above the knee amputation
A&OX3	Alert and oriented to person place and date
a&w	Alive and well
a-line	Arterial line
a-p	Anterior and posterior
a-p&lat	Anteroposterior and lateral
a-v	Atrioventricular
a/n or abnl	Abnormal
a/o	Alert and oriented

(Continued)

Medical Abbreviation	Term
AAA	Abdominal aortic aneurysm
ABG	Arterial blood gas
AC	Before eating or meal
ACLS	Advanced cardiac life support
ad lib	Ad libitim
ADAT	Advance diet as tolerated
AEA	Above elbow amputation
AF	Atrial fibrillation
Afl or a flutter	Atrial flutter
Agit	Agitation
AHHD	Arteriosclerotic hypertensive heart disease
AICD	Automatic implanted cardiac defibrillator
AIDS	Acquired immune deficiency syndrome
AIMI	Anteroinferior myocardial infarction
AIVR	Accelerated idioventricular rhythm
AKA	Above the knee amputation
Amb	Ambulate
AODM	Adult onset diabetes mellitus
Appt	Appointment
Apw	Aortopulmonary window
ARDS	Acute respiratory distress syndrome
ARF	Acute renal failure
AS	Aortic stenosis
ASAP	As soon as possible
ASCVD or ASCVHD	Atherosclerotic cardiovascular disease
ASD	Atrial septal defect
ASHD	Atherosclerotic heart disease
ASHVD	Atherosclerotic hypertensive vascular disease
ASMI	Anteroseptal myocardial infaction

ASVD	Arteriorsclerotic vascular disease
ASVHD	Arteriosclerotic vascular heart disease
AVS	Arteriovenous shunt
AV	Atrioventricular
AWMI	Anterior wall myocardial infarction
B	
BBB	Bundle branch block
BID	Twice a day
bil	Bilateral
BKA	Below the knee amputation
BP or b/p	Blood pressure
BPM	Beats per minute
BRP	Bathroom privileges
BS	Bowel or breath sounds
BW	Body weight
Bx	Biopsy
C	
c̄	With
C&S	Culture and sensitivity
CA	Cancer
CABG	Coronary artery bypass graft
CAD	Coronary artery disease
CAT	Computerized axial tomography
CBC	Complete blood count
CBG	Capillary blood gas
CC	Chief complaint
CCU	Cardiac care unit
CF	Cystic fibrosis
CHB	Complete heart block
CHF	Congestive heart failure

(Continued)

Medical Abbreviation	Term
CI	Cardiac index
CNS	Central nervous system
CO	Cardiac output
c/o	Complaining of
COLD	Chronic obstructive lung disease
COPD	Chronic obstructive pulmonary disease
CP	Chest pain
CPAP	Continuous positive airway pressure
CPK	Creatine phosphokinase
CPK-mb	Creatine phosphokinase myocardial band
CPR	Cardiopulmonary resuscitation
CRF	Chronic renal failure
CT	Computerized tomography
CVA	Cerebrovascular accident
CVC	Central venous catheter
CVHD	Cardiovascular heart disease
CVP	Central venous pressure
CXR	Chest x-ray
D	
DAT	Diet as tolerated
DC	Discontinue or discharge
DDx	Differential diagnosis
D5W	5% dextrose in water
DI	Diabetes insipidus
DIC	Disseminated intravascular coagulopathy
DIG	Digoxin
DJD	Degenerative joint disease

DKA	Diabetic ketoacidosis
DM	Diabetes mellitus
DNR	Do not resuscitate
DOA	Dead on arrival
d/s	Discharge summary
DOB	Date of birth
DOD	Date of discharge
DOE	Dyspnea on exertion
DTR	Deep tendon reflexes
DVT	Deep venous thrombosis
DX or Dx	Diagnosis
E	
EBL	Estimated blood loss
ECG or EKG	Electrocardiogram
ET	Endotracheal
ETT	Endotracheal tube
ETOH	Ethanol
Eval	Evaluation
F	
FBS	Fasting blood sugar
FEV	Forced expiratory volume
FTT	Failure to thrive
FU	Follow-up
FUO	Fever of unknown origin
fekg	Fetal electrocardiogram
fem pop, fem-pop, or fem/pop	Femoral popliteal
Fx	Fracture

(Continued)

Medical Abbreviation	Term
G	
GI	Gastrointestinal
Gr	Grain; 1 grain = 60 to 65 mg
GSW	Gun shot wound
gt or gtt	Drops
GTT	Glucose tolerance test
GU	Genitourinary
GXT	Graded exercise tolerance (stress test)
H	
HA	Headache
HAV	Hepatitis A virus
HBP	High blood pressure
HCT	Hematocrit
HDL	High density lipoprotein
HEENT	Head, eyes, ears, nose, throat
Hep A	Hepatitis A
Hep B	Hepatitis B
Hep lock or hep-lock	Heparin lock
Hgb	Hemoglobin
H/H	Hemoglobin/hematocrit
HIV	Human immunodeficiency virus
HO	History of
HOB	Head of bed
HOH	Hard of hearing
HPI	History of present illness
HR	Heart rate
HS	At bedtime
HSV	Herpes simplex virus
HTN	Hypertension
Hx	History

I	
I&D	Incision and drainage
IASD	Interatrial septal defect
I&O	Intake and output
ICS	Intercostal space
ICU	Intensive care unit
IPPB	Intermittent positive pressure breathing
ID	Infectious disease or identification
IDDM	Insulin dependent diabetes mellitus
IHSS	Idiopathic hypertropic subaortic stenosis
IM	Intramuscular
IMCU	Intermediate medical care unit
IMV	Intermittent mandatory ventilation
INF	Intravenous nutritional fluid
IPPB	Intermittent positive pressure breathing
IRBBB	Incomplete right bundle branch block
IRDM	Insulin resistant diabetes mellitus
ITP	Idiopathic thrombocytopenic purpua
IV	Intravenous
IVC	Inferior vena cava
IVP	Intravenous pyleogram
IWMI	Inferior wall myocardial infarction
J	
JODM	Juvenile onset diabetes mellitus
JVD	Jugular venous distention
K	
KOR	Keep open rate
KVO	Keep vein open

(Continued)

Medical Abbreviation	Term
L	
L	Left
LAD	Left axis deviation or left anterior descending
LAE	Left atrial enlargement
LAHB	Left anterior hemiblock
LAP	Left atrial pressure
LBBB	Left bundle branch block
LLL	Left lower lobe
LMP	Last menstrual period
LOC	Loss of consciousness or level of consciousness
LP	Lumbar puncture
LPN	Licensed practical nurse
LUL	Left upper lobe
LUQ	Left upper quadrant
LV	Left ventricle
LVAD	Left ventricular assist device
LVEDP	Left ventricular end diastolic pressure
LVF	Left ventricular failure
LVH	Left ventricular hypertrophy
LWMI	Lateral wall myocardial infarction
M	
MAP	Mean arterial pressure
MAST	Medical antishock trousers
MI	Myocardial infarction or mitral insufficiency
mL	Milliliter
mm	Millimeter
MLE	Midline episiotomy

MRI	Magnetic resonance imaging
MRSA	Methicillin-resistant *Staphylococcus aureus*
msec	Millisecond
MSSA	Methicillin-sensitive *Staphylococcus aureus*
MVA	Motor vehicle accident
N	
n&v, n + v, or n/v	Nausea and vomiting
n/a	Not applicable
NAD	No active disease
NAS	No added salt
NCV	Nerve conduction velocity
NED	No evidence of recurrent disease
NG	Nasogastric
NGT	Nasogastric tube
NIDDM	Non-insulin dependent diabetes mellitus
NKA	No known allergies
NKDA	No known drug allergies
NMR	Nuclear magnetic resonance
NPO	Nothing by mouth
NRM	No regular medication
NSAID	Non-steroidal anti-inflammatory drugs
NSR	Normal sinus rhythm
NT	Nasotracheal
NTG	Nitroglycerine
O	
OD	Overdose or right eye
OOB	Out of bed
OR	Operating room

(Continued)

Medical Abbreviation	Term
P	
P	Para
PA	Posteroanterior
PAC	Premature atrial contraction
PaO$_2$	Peripheral arterial oxygen content
PAP	Pulmonary artery pressure
PAT	Paroxysmal atrial tachycardia
PC	After eating
PCWP	Pulmonary capillary wedge pressure
PDA	Patent ductus arteriosus
PDR	*Physicians' Desk Reference*
PE	Pulmonary embolus, or physical exam, or pleural effusion
PEEP	Positive end expiratory pressure
PFT	Pulmonary function tests
PI	Pulmonic insufficiency disease
PMH	Previous medical history
PMI	Point of maximal impulse
PND	Paroxysmal nocturnal dyspnea
Pneumo	Pneumothorax
PO	By mouth
POD	Post-op day
PP	Postprandial
PR	By rectum
PRBC	Packed red blood cells
Pre-op or preop	Preoperative
PRN	As needed
PS	Pulmonic stenosis
PSVT	Paroxysmal supraventricular tachycardia
PT	Prothrombin time or physical therapy

Pt	Patient
PTCA	Percutaneous transluminal coronary angioplasty
PTT	Partial thromboplastin time
PUD	Peptic ulcer disease
PVC	Premature ventricular contraction
PVD	Peripheral vascular disease
PVI	Peripheral vascular insufficiency
PVT	Paroxysmal ventricular tachycardia
PEMI	Posterior wall myocardial infarction
PWP	Pulmonary wedge pressure
Q	
q	Every
qh	Every hour
q4h, q6h, . . .	Every 4 hours, every 6 hours, etc.
qid	Four times a day
QNS	Quantity not sufficient
R	
R	Right
RA	Rheumatoid arthritis or right atrium
RAD	Right atrial axis deviation
RAE	Right atrial enlargement
RAP	Right atrial pressure
RBBB	Right bundle branch block
RBC	Red blood cell
RDA	Recommended daily allowance
RLL	Right lower lobe
RML	Right middle lobe
R/O	Rule out
ROM	Range of motion

(Continued)

Medical Abbreviation	Term
ROS	Review of systems
RRR	Regular rate and rhythm
RT	Respiratory or radiation therapy
r/t	Related to
RTC	Return to clinic
RUL	Right upper lobe
RV	Residual volume
RVH	Right ventricular hypertrophy
Rx	Treatment
Rxn	Reaction
S	
s̄	Without
ss	One-half
s/s	Signs and symptoms
SA	Sinoatrial
SBE	Subacute bacterial endocarditis
SEM	Systolic ejection murmur
SG	Swan-Ganz
SGA	Small for gestational age
SICU	Surgical intensive care unit
sig	Write on label
SIMV	Synchronous intermittent mandatory ventilation
sl	Sublingual
SOAP	Subjective, objective, assessment, plan
SOB	Shortness of breath
SR	Sinus rhythm
Sub-Q, Sub Q	Subcutaneous
ST	Sinus tachycardia

stat	Immediate
SVT	Supraventricular tachycardia
Synch	Synchronized
Syst	Systolic
Sx	Symptoms
T	
TB	Tuberculosis
TIA	Transient ischemic attack
tid	Three times a day
TKO	To keep open
TLC	Total lung capacity
TNTC	Too numerous to count
TO	Telephone order
TPN	Total parentel nutrition
TV	Tidal volume
tw	Twice a week
TX	Treatment, transplant
U	
ud	As directed
UGI	Upper gastrointestinal
URI	Upper respiratory infection
US	Ultrasound
V	
V1	Chest lead I
V2	Chest lead II
V3	Chest lead III
V4	Chest lead IV
V5	Chest lead V

(Continued)

Medical Abbreviation	Term
V6	Chest lead VI
VC	Vital capacity
VO	Verbal or voice order
V/Q	Ventilation-perfusion
VS	Vital signs
VSS	Vital signs stable
VT	Ventricular tachycardia
VF or vfib	Ventricular fibrillation
W	
WD	Well developed
WF	White female
WM	White male
WN	Well nourished
WNL	Within normal limits
WPW	Wolff-Parkinson-White
X	
XRT	X-ray therapy
Y	
yo	Years old

DO NOT USE Abbreviations, Acronyms, and Symbols

Official Do Not Use List by JCAHO (Joint Commission Accreditation Hospital Organization) in 2004

Abbreviation	Potential Problem	Preferred Term
U (for unit)	Mistaken as zero, four, or cc.	Write "unit."
IU (for international unit)	Mistaken as IV (intravenous) or 10 (ten)	Write "international unit."
Q.D., Q.O.D.	Mistaken for each other. The period after the Q can be mistaken for an "I" and the "O" can be mistaken for "I"	Write "daily" and "every other day."
Trailing zero (X.0 mg), Lack of leading zero (.X mg)	Decimal point is missed	Never write a zero by itself after a decimal point (X mg), and always use a zero before a decimal point (0.X mg).
MS MSO_4 $MgSO_4$	Confused for one another. Can mean morphine sulfate or magnesium sulfate	Write "morphine sulfate" or "magnesium sulfate."

Additional Abbreviations, Acronyms, and Symbols to Be Included in the Future Lists

Abbreviation	Potential Problem	Preferred Term
> (greater than) < (less than)	Misinterpreted as the number "7" (seven) or the letter "L"	Write "greater than." Write "less than."
Abbreviations for drug names	Misinterpreted due to similar abbreviations for multiple drugs	Write drug names in full.
Apothecary units	Unfamiliar to many practitioners Confused with metric unit	Use metric units.
@	Mistaken for the number "2" (two)	Write "at."
μg (for microgram)	Mistaken for mg (milligrams) resulting in one-thousand-fold dosing overdose	Write "mcg."
c.c. (for cubic centimeter)	Mistaken for U (units) when poorly written	Write "ml" for milliliters.
H.S. (for half-strength or Latin abbreviation for bedtime)	Mistaken for either half-strength or hour of sleep (at bedtime) q.H.S. mistaken for every hour. All can result in a dosing error.	Write out "half-strength" or "at bedtime."
T.I.W. (for three times a week)	Mistaken for three times a day or twice weekly resulting in an overdose	Write "3 times weekly" or "three times weekly."

S.C. or S.Q. (for subcutaneous)	Mistaken as SL for sublingual, or "5 every"	Write "Sub-Q," "subQ," or "subcutaneously."
D/C (for discharge)	Interpreted as discontinue whatever medications follow (typically discharge meds)	Write "discharge."
A.S., A.D., A.U. (Latin abbreviation for left, right, or both ears) O.S., O.D., O.U., (Latin abbreviation for left, right, or both eyes)	Mistaken for each other (e.g., AS for OS, AD for OD, AU for OU, etc.)	Write "left ear," "right ear," or "both ears"; "left eye," "right eye," or "both eyes."

Appendix D

Answer Key

Chapter One

Checkpoint Question 1-1

1. Cardiovascular disease

Checkpoint Question 1-2

1. Dr. Augusta D. Waller

Checkpoint Question 1-3

1. Records the ECG tracing, prepares the tracing for the physician's interpretation, and determines if ECG tracing is accurate without artifact

Troubleshooting: Remain Calm

1. Say: "The physician would like me to do a recording of your heart." Do not show signs of fear or anxiety. Remain calm during the procedure.

Checkpoint Questions 1-4

1. Hospitals, clinics, doctors' offices and by emergency personnel in the community
2. Sudden cardiac arrest, ventricular fibrillation, and ventricular tachycardia without a pulse

Troubleshooting: Consent

1. A family member or a witness, but the patient should write an X if possible.

Checkpoint Question 1-5

1. Follow universal and standard precautions.

Chapter Review

(Match)

1. f	5. a
2. b	6. g
3. d	7. e
4. c	

True

8. False: An ECG machine does not produce electricity; it only records the electrical activity of the heart.
9. True
10. True
11. False: A transtelephonic monitor transmits an ECG over the telephone line.

Multiple Choice

12. b	20. c
13. b	21. b
14. a	22. a
15. d	23. d
16. d	24. b
17. a	25. b
18. b	26. d
19. b	27. a

What Should You Do? *Critical Thinking Application*

28. Your favorite uncle should have an ECG as part of a routine physical since he is over 40; however, the physician should order this. You should not perform an ECG on someone without a

verbal or written order. You may, however, practice an ECG on someone as long as the individual understands you are not going to interpret it or use it for diagnosis.

29. "Mr. Smith, I am not trained to interpret the results of your ECG. As soon as the physician sees it, I am sure he or she will discuss the results with you. How are you feeling right now? Are you having any discomfort or pain? How would you rate your pain on a scale of 1 to 10, with 1 being the least pain and 10 being the most pain?"

30. Every patient has the right to privacy. Your co-worker may have just forgotten to close the door and/or drape the patient. You could quietly close the door or curtain in order to provide for privacy. It would be best not to make any statement or comment to your co-worker at this time unless he or she asks.

31. You should tell your supervisor how you feel and explain the need to go to the restroom. Do not leave the monitors unattended except for extreme or severe circumstances. You should find someone to view the monitors when you are not there. You have a legal and ethical responsibility to ensure that someone is watching the monitors when you are not there. Hopefully, your supervisor will be able to find someone to take your place in order for you to go home.

Chapter Two

Checkpoint Questions 2-1

1. The process of transporting blood to and from the body tissues.
2. The electrical activity of the heart.

Checkpoint Questions 2-2

1. Myocardium
2. Bicuspid or mitral valve

Checkpoint Question 2-3

1. Coronary arteries

Checkpoint Question 2-4

1. When the blood leaves right ventricles and travels to the lungs, when the heart muscle contracts, and when the blood leaves left ventricles to body via aorta.

Checkpoint Questions 2-5

1. Excitability
2. AV node

Checkpoint Questions 2-6

1. Depolarization
2. P wave

Chapter Review

Matching

1. d		6. f
2. i		7. g
3. e		8. b
4. a		9. h
5. j		10. c

Matching II

11. g		16. e
12. b		17. a
13. c		18. j
14. i		19. h
15. f		20. d

Multiple Choice

21. b
22. c
23. d
24. a
25. a
26. c
27. a
28. c
29. b
30. d

Matching III

31. c
32. a
33. h
34. b
35. f
36. e
37. d
38. g

Label the Parts

39.

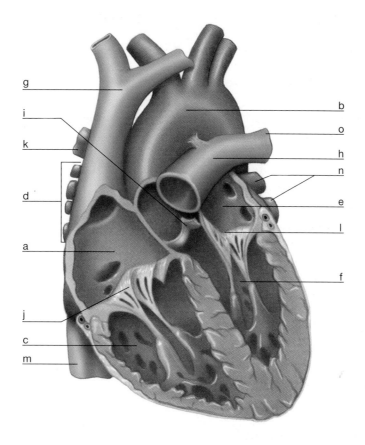

40.

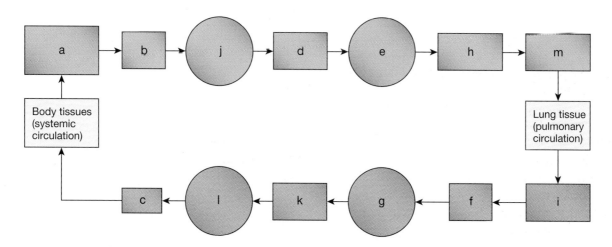

41.

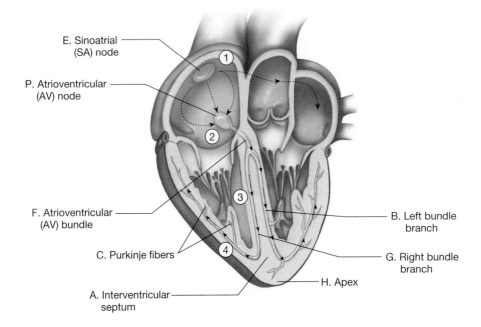

- E. Sinoatrial (SA) node — ①
- P. Atrioventricular (AV) node — ②
- F. Atrioventricular (AV) bundle
- C. Purkinje fibers
- A. Interventricular septum
- B. Left bundle branch
- G. Right bundle branch
- H. Apex
- ③
- ④

42.

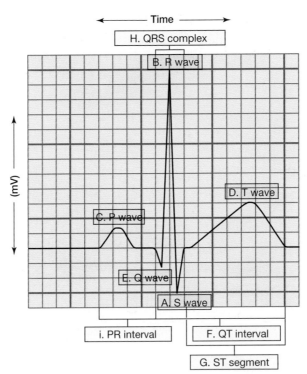

- Time
- H. QRS complex
- B. R wave
- (mV)
- D. T wave
- C. P wave
- E. Q wave
- A. S wave
- i. PR interval
- F. QT interval
- G. ST segment

Right or Wrong?

43. a. Incorrect: "The valves between the atria and the ventricles are atrioventricular."

b. Incorrect: "The ventricles always pump the blood"

c. Correct

d. Incorrect: "The coronary arteries carry oxygenated blood."

e. Incorrect: "The pulmonary artery carries deoxygenated blood"

f. Correct

g. Incorrect: "In general, if you are a man you will have a slower heartbeat."

h. Incorrect: "The top chambers of the heart are the atria, and the bottom chambers of the heart are the ventricles."

i. Incorrect: "The left ventricle is sometimes known as the workhorse of the heart."

j. Correct

Voyage Through the Heart

44. a. superior vena cava
   b. tricuspid
   c. pulmonary veins
   d. left atrium
   e. coronary arteries

What Should You Do? *Critical Thinking Application*

45. The atrioventricular (AV) node is responsible for slowing the electrical conduction from the atria to the ventricles. This delay in electrical conduction prevents all of the electrical impulses from stimulating the ventricles.

46. The sympathetic branch of the autonomic nervous system responded to the stress from the darkness and sound and increased your and your patient's heart rates. Without further stimulation, your and your patient's heart rates will return to normal. It would be best to wait for awhile until the heart rate is within normal limits before recording the ECG.

Chapter Three

Checkpoint Question 3-1

1. The equipment and lead system

Troubleshooting: Check the Lead Wires

1. Recheck the lead wires to make sure they are placed correctly.

Checkpoint Questions 3-2

1. 10 leads
2. aVL, aVR, aVF

Troubleshooting: Changing the ECG Tracing Speed

1. Mark the tracing as shown here. Notify the health care provider who will be interpreting the tracing, if possible.

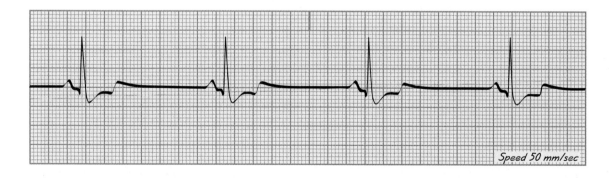

Speed 50 mm/sec

Troubleshooting: Changing the Gain

1. Increase or adjust the gain.

Checkpoint Questions 3-3

1. Three leads
2. Rhythm rate is too fast, can't clearly identify waves because they are too close together, per physician's orders

Checkpoint Question 3-4

1. Silver disposable electrodes

Troubleshooting: Handle the ECG Report with Care

1. Bring the location of the report to the physician's attention or remove the charts and place on top to protect the ECG recording from damage.

Troubleshooting: Counting the Heart Rate

1. Seven complexes; estimated heart rate 70 beats per minute.

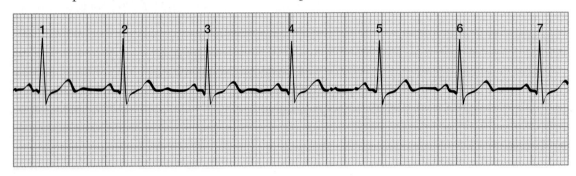

Checkpoint Question 3-5

1. 300 boxes per minute

Chapter Review

Matching

1. c	4. a	7. c	10. a
2. b	5. b	8. c	11. c
3. a	6. c	9. b	12. c

Matching II

13. j	16. b	19. g	22. a
14. k	17. e	20. d	23. h
15. c	18. f	21. i	

Multiple Choice

24. a	28. a	32. a	36. a
25. b	29. d	33. c	
26. c	30. a	34. c	
27. b	31. c	35. d	

Matching III

37. a
38. c
39. b

Matching IV

40. d
41. b
42. a
43. c

Label the Parts

44.

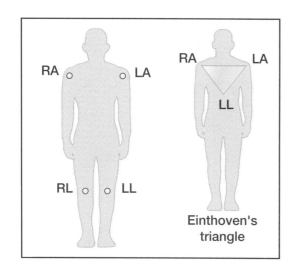 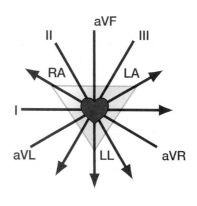

45.

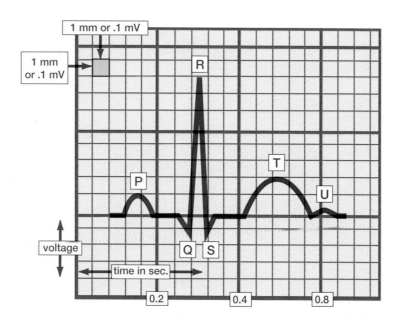

46. Boxes between R waves—3. 300 ÷ 3 = Rate of 100 beats per minute

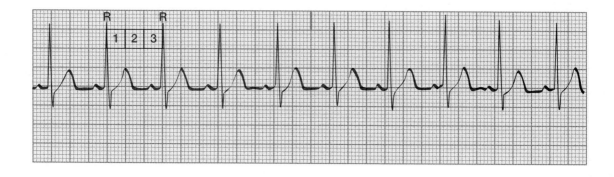

47. Large boxes between R waves—1.5. Rate 300 ÷ 1.5 = 200 beats per minute

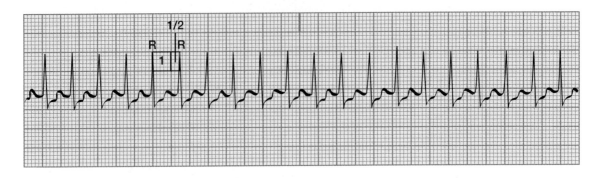

48. 14 complete complexes × 10 = 140 beats per minute

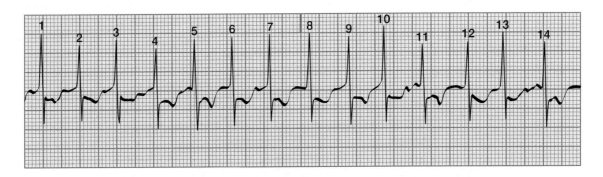

49. Four complexes × 10 = 40 beats per minute

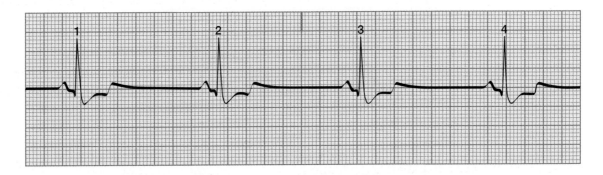

50. 16 small squares between 2 R waves 1500 ÷ 16 = 93.75 or 94 beats per minute

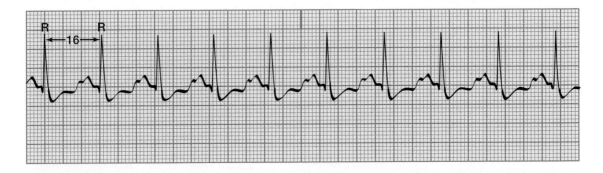

51. 26 small boxes between R waves 1500 ÷ 26 = 57.69 or 58 beats per minute

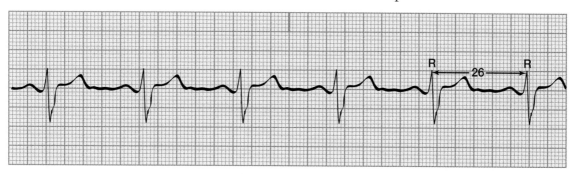

What Should You Do? *Critical Thinking Application*

52. The machine is about to run out of paper. You should change the paper before performing the next ECG.

53. ECG electrodes dry out. Check to see if the bag has been properly sealed. If so, you may use them if they do not appear to be dried out. Otherwise, it is best that you use new electrodes. If you attempt to use the electrodes after you determine they have been properly sealed but you have difficulty with the tracing, you still may need to replace them.

54. You have probably attached the lead wires incorrectly. Check each lead color and make sure the leads are properly placed. Since you cannot read the letters, refer to the manufacturer's directions to identify the correct color for each lead wire.

55. Check the machine for a stylus control. Turn the heat down on the stylus so the line is thinner. Make sure the machine is standardized if that is required of the machine you are using. When using a newer ECG machine, you may want to check the LCD display. The machine may identify the problem for you. In addition, if one of the leads does not record properly, you will need to repeat the tracing. Use the lead selector to repeat the entire 12-lead ECG procedure. In general, you should be familiar with the controls of the machine you are using. Review the manufacturer's directions carefully.

Chapter Four

Checkpoint Question 4-1

1. The experience should be pleasant, it should not produce anxiety, it must be done correctly, and the tracing must be accurate.

Checkpoint Question 4-2

1. Name, birth date, identification number or medical record number, age, sex, race, current cardiac medication being taken, weight and height, special condition or position of the patient.

Checkpoint Question 4-3

1. Indicate to the patient you are providing for his or her privacy during the procedure.

Checkpoint Questions 4-4

1. Midaxillary line

2. It is a ridge about an inch below the suprasternal notch where the main part of the sternum and the manubrium attach.

Troubleshooting: The Midclavicular Line

1. The midclavicular line may not run through the nipple line; use the clavicle as the landmark, not the nipple.

Checkpoint Question 4-5

1. Check the manufacturer's directions in the operator's manual for optimum connection techniques.

Checkpoint Questions 4-6

1. Refer to Table 4-4.

2. Refer to Table 4-5.

Checkpoint Question 4-7

1. 8 to 10 inches

Troubleshooting: Multiple ECGs

1. On the same or as close as possible to the sites previously used. Look for marks on the chest.

Troubleshooting: Handling a Flatline Tracing

1. Check the patient first. If the patient responds, check the lead wires, electrodes, and cables. If the patient does not respond, treat the emergency.

Checkpoint Questions 4-8

1. Body tremor
2. Too loose or incorrect electrode application; old or dried out electrode gel or solution; oil, lotion, or dirt under the electrodes, or pulling on the electrodes from unsupported lead wires.

Checkpoint Questions 4-9

1. Results should be given immediately to your supervisor or the physician, and a printed copy is placed on top of the chart.
2. Cut the tracing into smaller segments to place on the preprinted mount, mount the tracing before it is evaluated, and mark each lead appropriately.

Checkpoint Question 4-10

1. So that the ECG machine is available to record a tracing; so that the equipment is in good condition at all times and will not transmit diseases to other patients.

Checkpoint Questions 4-11

1. Their fast heart rates make the tracing difficult to evaluate.
2. Document the change on the ECG tracing.

Checkpoint Question 4-12

1. Record the first 12 leads with all the leads in normal position, record the second 12 leads with the chest leads moved to new positions, and indicate on the second 12 leads the new lead labels.

Checkpoint Question 4-13

1. Record the ECG tracing after the patient's seizure has stopped, protect the patient from harm, and call for help.

Chapter Review

Matching

1. d
2. b
3. c
4. a
5. e
6. b
7. f
8. d
9. a
10. c
11. c
12. b
13. a

Multiple Choice

14. a
15. a
16. c
17. d
18. b
19. d
20. b
21. b
22. c
23. c
24. a
25. a
26. a
27. a
28. c
29. b
30. a
31. b
32. d
33. a

True/False

34. True
35. True
36. False: Personal protective equipment should be worn during an ECG based upon the patient's condition and/or disease.

Matching II

37. d
38. g
39. k
40. m
41. h
42. a
43. e
44. l
45. b
46. i
47. f
48. c
49. n
50. j

Identification

51.
   1. manubrium
   2. angle of Louis
   3. suprasternal notch
   4. clavicles
   5. fourth ICS
   6. fifth ICS
   7. midclavicular line
   8. anterior axillary line
   9. midaxillary line

52.
   a. V1—fourth intercostal space, right sternal border
   b. V2—fourth intercostal space, left sternal border
   c. V3—halfway between V2 and V4
   d. V4—fifth intercostal space at the midclavicular line

e. V5—on the same horizontal level with V4, at the anterior axillary line

f. V6—on the same horizontal level with V4 and V5, at the midaxillary line

What Should You Do? *Critical Thinking Application*

53. Do not panic. Check the patient to make sure he or she is breathing and has a pulse. If so, you will need to check all of your electrodes and lead wires for proper connection. If the patient is not breathing or does not have a pulse, report a Code Blue and initiate CPR immediately.

54. Parkinson's disease produces fine tremors. The patient is probably experiencing somatic tremor. You may have the patient place the hands palms down under the buttocks to reduce the tremor. If the tremor is still noticeable, you should note on the tracing that the patient has Parkinson's disease.

55. Report this to your supervisor immediately. If instructed, complete the ECG procedure, observing the patient carefully. Note on the ECG that the patient was experiencing chest pains during the procedure.

56. Explain to the patient that you are not allowed to give a copy and he or she should ask the physician for a copy.

Chapter Five

Checkpoint Question 5-1

1. Waves, segments, and intervals on the ECG tracing

Checkpoint Questions 5-2

1. Rhythm, rate, P wave configuration, PR interval measurement, and QRS duration and configuration

2. 70 beats per minute

3. Are all the QRS complexes of equal length? What is the actual measurement, and is it within normal limits? Do all QRS complexes look alike, and are the unusual QRS complexes associated with an ectopic beat?

Troubleshooting: Report the Patient Condition, Not the Tracing

1. Report the situation to your supervisor immediately. The patient is showing signs of decreased cardiac output, which includes pale skin and respiratory difficulty.

Checkpoint Questions 5-3

1. Sinus rhythm

2. Bradycardia has a heart rate of less than 60. Tachycardia has a heart rate of greater than 100.

3. Sinus dysrhythmia

Troubleshooting: Sinus Arrest

1. Asystole is considered a life-threatening dysrhythmia that requires immediate CPR. You should follow the facility policy for a cardiac arrest sometimes called a Code Blue.

Checkpoint Questions 5-4

1. If the PACs are frequent, you would expect the patient to have symptoms of low cardiac output.

2. Oxygen therapy and careful monitoring to watch for the rhythm to change to sinus rhythm or progress to atrial fibrillation

3. Chaotic disorganized activity between QRS complexes

4. MAT is considered more serious because it is usually caused by an underlying disease such as emphysema, CHF, or acute mitral valve regurgitation. WAP is a common occurrence in children, older adults, and well-conditioned athletes.

Checkpoint Question 5-5

1. A junctional rhythm has a rate atrial and ventricular of 40 to 60 beats per minute. A PJC rate will be based upon the underlying rhythm. A junctional rhythm has P-P and R-R intervals that are regular and similar. A PJC typically has an irregular rhythm.

Checkpoint Questions 5-6

1. The rate is usually over 150 beats per minute, and the origination point is from an ectopic focus originating above the ventricles, in the atria, or junctional region of the heart.

2. Increase the paper speed so the licensed practitioner may be able to analyze the tracing more carefully.

3. Sinus tachycardia, atrial flutter, atrial fibrillation, junctional tachycardia

Troubleshooting: Mobitz I Versus Mobitz II

1. For a Mobitz I (Wenckebach), the PR interval in front of the dropped QRS complex will be longer than the PR interval after the dropped QRS complex.

Checkpoint Questions 5-7

1. First degree AV block, second degree AV block, Mobitz I (Wenckebach), second degree AV block, Mobitz II, and third degree or complete heart block. Complete heart block is most serious.

2. In Mobitz I, the PR interval in front of the dropped QRS complex will be longer than the PR interval after the dropped QRS complex. This rhythm usually resolves itself. The Mobitz II the PR interval in front of and behind the dropped QRS complex will be constant. This is a critical condition.

3. Observe the patient for signs of low cardiac output. The patient may be unconscious. Contact the licensed practitioner most often by initiating a Code Blue. A pacemaker may be inserted, and the rhythm strips should be mounted and identified in the patient's medical record.

Checkpoint Questions 5-8

1. The electrical activity cannot travel down the bundle branch and a bundle branch block occurs.

2. RBBB: The impulse travels to the bundle of His normally, then down the left bundle branch to activate the left ventricle; then the current travels to the right ventricle. LBBB: The impulse travels down the right bundle branch and the right ventricle contracts; then the impulse travels to the left ventricle activating the septum in an abnormal right-to-left fashion.

Troubleshooting: Escape Beats

1. Heart rate of 46 beats per minute

Checkpoint Questions 5-9

1. An idioventricular rhythm has a rate of 20 to 40 beats per minute and an accelerated idioventricular rhythm has a rate of 40 to 100 beats per minute.

2. Both rhythms are life-threatening and will require basic and advanced life support.

3. Ventricular tachycardia has three or more PVCs and a rate of greater than 100 beats per minute. Ventricular fibrillation is chaotic electrical activity with only fibrillatory waves.

Checkpoint Question 5-10

1. Malfunction—failure to pace; malsensing—failure to sense; loss of capture—failure to depolarize; and oversensing—perceiving electrical current impulses from sources other than the heart.

Chapter Review

Matching I

1 j	5. e	9. f
2. h	6. d	10. g
3. c	7. b	
4. i	8. a	

It's Your Choice

11. a	21. c
12. b	22. b
13. d	23. a
14. a	24. d
15. c	25. a
16. c	26. d
17. b	27. d
18. b	28. d
19. d	29. a
20. b	30. b

Matching II

31. h	35. g
32. c	36. f
33. d	37. b
34. e	38. a

What Should You Do? *Critical Thinking Application*

39. First, determine if the chaotic activity is due to artifact. Troubleshoot for artifact using the methods described in Chapter 3. Check the electrodes and lead wires as your first step. If you determine it is not artifact, check the patient. Talk to him and observe for signs of low cardiac output. If you cannot correct the tracing by troubleshooting for artifact or you observe signs of low cardiac output, it might

be an abnormal rhythm such as atrial fibrillation. Report abnormalities immediately to the licensed practitioner.

40. Second degree atrioventricular block, Mobitz II, is more serious than Mobitz I. Mobitz I is a temporary condition, whereas Mobitz II is a chronic condition due to damage to the atrioventricular node.

41 It is essential that the patient's cardiac output parameters be observed for level of consciousness. Some patients will remain conscious and other patients will be unconscious when experiencing ventricular tachycardia. The level of consciousness determines whether a Code Blue is initiated or not.

42 Mr. Green needs to be monitored in an MCL I lead since the continuous monitoring equipment has three leads. This is done by placing the positive electrode in the fourth intercostal space to the right of the sternum border. The negative electrode is placed at the left shoulder region.

Mr Green could also be evaluated as to the location of the blockage with a 12-lead ECG recording. The evaluation of the blockage is determined when looking at the lead V1 for the characteristic patterns of either the RBBB or LBBB.

43. Observe the patient for signs and symptoms of low cardiac output. Any evidence of low cardiac output needs immediate notification to the licensed practitioner for appropriate treatment.

Rhythm Identification

44. Sinus rhythm
45. Sinus bradycardia
46. Sinus tachycardia
47. Sinus dysrhythmia
48. Premature atrial contractions
49. Atrial flutter
50. Atrial fibrillation
51. First degree atrioventricular block
52. Second degree atrioventricular block, Mobitz I (Wenckebach)
53. Second degree atrioventricular block, Mobitz II
54. Third degree atrioventricular block
55. Premature ventricular contractions
56. Ventricular tachycardia
57. Ventricular fibrillation
58. Asystole
59. Pacemaker rhythms

60. Rhythm: Ventricles regular
P wave: Cannot determine
QRS complex: Cannot determine

Rate: 71
PRI: Cannot determine
Interpretation: 60 cycle interference

61. Rhythm: V-tach-reg, V-fib-irreg.
P wave: Absent
QRS complex: Greater than 0.12 second

Rate: V-tach 167, V-fib-cannot determine
PRI: Cannot determine
Interpretation: Ventricular tachycardia
Paroxysmal ventricular
Fibrillation

62. Rhythm: Regular
P wave: Partially buried in "T" wave
QRS complex: _____

Rate: 143
PRI: Cannot determine
Interpretation: Sinus tachycardia

63. Rhythm: Regular
P wave: Rounded, upright with spike
QRS complex: 0.16 second

Rate: 83
PRI: 0.18 second
Interpretation: AV sequential paced rhythm

64. Rhythm: Regular
P wave: Absent
QRS complex: 0.22 second

Rate: 14
PRI: Absent
Interpretation: Agonal

65. Rhythm: Atrial-regular
               Ventricular-irreg
P wave: Rounded and upright
QRS complex: 0.08 second

Rate: Atrial-70, ventricles-60
PRI: Variable "cycle"
Interpretation: Mobitz second degree type I

66. Rhythm: Regular
P wave: Inverted
QRS complex: 0.06 second

Rate: 41
PRI: 0.08 second
Interpretation: Junctional escape rhythm

67. Rhythm: Irregular
P wave: Upright, inverted-early complex
QRS complex: 0.08 second

Rate: 70
PRI: 0.16 second
Interpretation: Sinus rhythm with PJCs

68. Rhythm: Regular
P wave: Rounded and upright
QRS complex: 0.08 second

Rate: 71
PRI: 0.16 second
Interpretation: Normal sinus rhythm

69. Rhythm: Regular
P wave: Rounded, upright w/ spike
QRS complex: 0.08 second

Rate: 75
PRI: 0.14 second
Interpretation: Atrial paced rhythm

70. Rhythm: Regular
P wave: Rounded and upright
QRS complex: 0.08 second

Rate: 71
PRI: 0.28 second
Interpretation: First degree heart block

71. Rhythm: Irregular
P wave: Rounded and upright
QRS complex: 0.08-underlying
               rhythm ventricular
               beats-greater than
               0.12 second

Rate: Atria-60 ventricles-80
PRI: 0.16 second
Interpretation: Sinus rhythm w/
               nonsustained run of
               ventricular tachycardia or
               salvo PVCs

72. Rhythm: Irregular
P wave: Absent, "f" waves
QRS complex: 0.08 second

Rate: Atria-Unable to determine ventricles-100
PRI: Cannot measure
Interpretation: Atrial fibrillation

73. Rhythm: Regular
P wave: Rounded and upright
QRS complex: 0.08 second

Rate: 36
PRI: 0.16 second
Interpretation: Sinus bradycardia

74. Rhythm: Irregular
P wave: Absent
QRS complex: Greater than 0.12 second

Rate: 70
PRI: Unable to measure
Interpretation: Ventricular paced rhythm w/
failure to capture

75. Rhythm: Regular
P wave: Rounded and upright
QRS complex: 0.08 second

Rate: Atria-107 ventricles-36
PRI: 0.14 second
Interpretation: Third degree (complete) heart block

76. Rhythm: Irregular
P wave: Absent "f" waves
QRS complex: 0.08 second

Rate: Ventricles-50
PRI: Absent
Interpretation: Atrial fibrillation

77. Rhythm: Regular
P wave: Absent
QRS complex: greater than 0.12 second

Rate: 36
PRI: Absent
Interpretation: Idioventricular rhythm

78. Rhythm: Regular
P wave: Inverted
QRS complex: 0.08 second

Rate: 71
PRI: 0.08 second
Interpretation: Accelerated junctional rhythm

79. Rhythm: Regular
P wave: Absent, "f" waves
QRS complex: 0.06 second

Rate: Atria-293 ventricles-73
PRI: Absent
Interpretation: Atrial flutter 4:1

80. Rhythm: Irregular
P wave: Round and upright
QRS complex: 0.08 second

Rate: 80
PRI: 0.16 second
Interpretation: Sinus rhythm w/ multifocal couplet PVCs

81. Rhythm: Irregular
P wave: Round and upright
QRS complex: 0.10 second

Rate: 70
PRI: 0.14 second
Interpretation: Sinus rhythm w/ PACs

82. Rhythm: Regular
P wave: Round and upright
QRS complex: _____

Rate: Atria-90 ventricles-36
PRI: Variable
Interpretation: Third degree (complete) heart block

83. Rhythm: Irregular
P wave: Round and upright
QRS complex: 0.08 second

Rate: 60
PRI: 0.16 second
Interpretation: Sinus rhythm w/ unifocal bigeminy PVCs

Chapter Six

Checkpoint Question 6-1
1. The testing does not require entrance into a body cavity, tissue, or blood vessel.

Checkpoint Question 6-2
1. Safety, education and preparation of the patient, attaching electrodes, instruction for reporting of patient symptoms, monitoring of blood pressure, and performing 12-lead ECG

Checkpoint Question 6-3
1. Cause of chest pain, functional capacity of the heart, heart disease, limitations for an exercise program, abnormal heart rhythms induced by exercise, and the effectiveness of heart medication

Checkpoint Question 6-4

1. Because the patient is not able to exercise or the physician wants images of the heart.

HIPAA, Law, and Ethics: Informed Consent

1. Since informed consent is mandatory, you must solve the problem before beginning the procedure. Start by identifying why the patient is resisting then use Table 6.2 possible solutions to troubleshoot the situation.

Checkpoint Question 6-5

1. Because of the risks and complications involved in the procedure

Checkpoint Question 6-6

1. Not everyone can have a standard stress test. Certain conditions that limit the patient include heart aneurysm, uncontrolled disturbances in the heartbeat, inflammation surrounding the heart or heart muscle, severe anemia, uncontrolled hypertension, unstable angina, or congestive heart failure.

Troubleshooting: Reporting Problems

1. Check the pulse and respiration and begin emergency procedures as appropriate.

Checkpoint Question 6-7

1. 103 to 145 beats per minute

Checkpoint Question 6-8

1. Rest for several hours, avoid extreme temperature, avoid stimulants, no hot shower or bath for 2 hours, discuss the results with the physician, up to 10 days after the test when available

Chapter Review

Multiple Choice

1. a	5. a
2. c	6. b
3. b	7. d
4. d	8. c

Patient Education

9. Incorrect: Patients should avoid alcohol, tobacco, and caffeine for at least 3 hours prior to exercise electrocardiography.
10. Correct
11. Correct
12. Incorrect: The physician should discuss the results of exercise electrocardiography with the patient as soon as the results are available.
13. Correct
14. Incorrect: Check the manufacturer's directions and the diagram provided with the test machine for correct placement of the leads for exercise electrocardiography.
15. Correct

16. **Lead Placement**

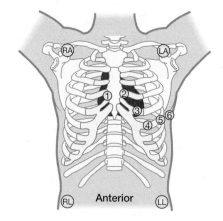

Matching

17. m	25. c
18. k	26. g
19. j	27. h
20. a	28. i
21. f	29. l
22. b	
23. d	
24. e	

True/False

30. False: An invasive procedure requires entrance into a body cavity, tissue, or blood vessel.

31. False: A Bruce Protocol is most commonly utilized for a stress test.

32. True

33. False: A 12-lead ECG is obtained toward the end of each stage of exercise electrocardiography.

34. True

35. True

What Should You Do? *Critical Thinking Application*

36. Since the chart does not indicate whether Mr. Rollins should omit any medications prior to exercise electrocardiography, you should check with the physician. Since Atenolol is a beta blocker, it is particularly important that you determine whether this medication should be taken. Ask the licensed practitioner or physician whether medication should be held on the day of the test. When asking, be certain to provide him or her with a list of all the medications Mr. Rollins is taking. If Mr. Rollins is in a hurry, you could obtain the answer and call him prior to the day of the test. However, if Mr. Rollins is not available by phone or the test is scheduled for the next day, you will need to inform him of the medication changes prior to leaving.

37. Determine whether the patient is responsive. If so, evaluate the patient including the blood pressure. Keep in mind that a physician will be present. If the patient is not responsive, provide cardiopulmonary resuscitation immediately. If CPR has already been started, obtain the emergency equipment and additional personnel to assist. A Code Blue or 911 emergency will be initiated.

38. After exercise electrocardiography, the patient is instructed to avoid extreme temperatures and tobacco. These things cause stress on the heart. Discuss this information with Mrs. Annon and encourage her to wait at least 2 hours before smoking and to remain inside the air-conditioned facility until her husband arrives.

39. You should explain to Mr. Wong that the thallium stress test requires 3 to 4 hours of his time and he should plan to miss work for at least one afternoon. Do not forget to explain to him the necessary preparation for the test.

Chapter Seven

Checkpoint Question 7-1

1. 24 to 48 hours

Checkpoint Question 7-2

1. Applying and removing the monitor, patient education, ensuring the placement of the results, scanning the tape or digital disk, distinguishing artifact

Checkpoint Question 7-3

1. The health care provider that interprets the results can compare the activities in the diary with the ECG tracing to help identify the cause of any abnormalities.

Troubleshooting: Patient Problems

1. Check the policy first, then have the patient press the electrode in place or return to your facility depending upon your policy.

Checkpoint Question 7-4

1. These patients are at an inpatient facility, and their activities and actions are already being monitored. They can report symptoms immediately, and their ECG tracing is being monitored as well.

Troubleshooting: Patient Instructions

1. Yes, activities should remain normal.

Checkpoint Question 7-5

1. For comfort and convenience, to reduce artifact, and to provide access to the chest.

Checkpoint Question 7-6

1. "Let me check with the licensed practitioner or supervisor to ensure that I answer this question correctly." or "Give me a second I will ask the doctor to be certain I answer correctly."

Checkpoint Question 7-7

1. Leads or wires become loose or detached or are pulling. The monitor, wires, or electrodes get wet.

Troubleshooting: No Diary

1. Ask the patient to return with the diary before removing the monitor.

Checkpoint Question 7-8

1. Improper lead attachment, incomplete patient diary, failure of patient to maintain normal routine

Chapter Review

Ordering

1. 4
2. 1
3. 3
4. 2
5. 13
6. 6
7. 10
8. 9
9. 5
10. 11
11. 12
12. 8
13. 7

Matching

14. d
15. g
16. h
17. e
18. i
19. f
20. c
21. a
22. b

Patient Education

23. Incorrect: The patient is instructed to participate in his or her normal activities during the monitoring
24. Correct
25. Incorrect: Mr. Booth should not take a tub bath or shower during the monitoring. He may take only sponge baths. The monitor should not get wet under any circumstance.
26. Correct
27. Incorrect: Patients should take their medications as normally scheduled unless specifically instructed not to by the physician.

Multiple Choice

28. c
29. d
30. b
31. b
32. a

Lead Placement

33. white - manubrium
34. red - centered over rib
35. green - centered over rib
36. brown - manobrium
37. black - V4/V5 area centered over rib

What Should You Do? *Critical Thinking Application*

38. Monitors are expensive and easily damaged. The first thing you should do is examine the monitor for obvious cracks or breaks. If you do not find any damage, insert the batteries and test to see if it functions properly. If it does not work, you may need to contact the manufacturer for repair. Most importantly, you should report the incident to your supervisor and use a different monitor for ambulatory monitoring while the original monitor is being serviced.

39. It appears that your patient was not given the proper instructions, did not understand the instructions, or was unable or unwilling to write in the diary. You can question the patient to see if he or she remembers some of the activities during the 24- to 48-hour period and attempt to fill in the blanks. You would need to make note of this on the diary. You may want to show the physician or your supervisor the diary to determine if the monitoring should be repeated or continued. It may be wise to do this prior to removing the monitor, in case the physician decides to continue the monitoring. Most importantly, if the monitoring is going to occur again, you should ensure that the patient understands and is able to complete the diary. Proper patient education is important. You may also be able to enlist the help of a family member if the patient is unable or unwilling to complete the diary.

40. For some reason, Mr. Hernandez is not willing to complete the diary. Try to understand his reason by discussing it with him. Ask him questions to gain a better understanding of the problem. He may be illiterate or just uncooperative. In either case, you will need to enlist the cooperation of a family member to ensure that the diary is complete. Certainly ambulatory monitoring will not be effective unless the patient completes the diary.

41. When the ambulatory monitor is in place, the patient is instructed to avoid magnets, metal detectors, high-voltage areas, and electric blankets. At the airport, all individuals are required to walk through a metal detector before they can enter the gate area. While Ms. Lin can still go the airport, she should not walk through this metal detector.

Glossary

A

AC (alternating current) interference Unwanted markings on the ECG caused by other electrical current sources.

ambulate To walk.

angina Pain around the heart radiating to the arm, caused by lack of oxygen to the heart muscle.

angiogram An invasive procedure during which x-rays are taken of a blood vessel after injection of a radiopaque substance.

angioplasty Surgical repair of blood vessels.

angle of Louis A ridge about an inch or so below the suprasternal notch where the main part of the sternum and the top of the sternum, known as the manubrium, are attached.

anterior axillary line An imaginary vertical line starting at the edge of the chest where the armpit begins.

anti-arrhythmic Type of medication given to prevent arrhythmias.

aorta The largest artery of the body, which transports blood from the left ventricle of the heart to the entire body.

aortic semilunar valve Valve located in the aorta that prevents the backflow of blood into the left ventricle.

apnea The absence of breathing

arrhythmia Abnormal or absence of normal heartbeat, also known as *dysrhythmia*.

artifact Unwanted marks on the ECG tracing caused by activity other than the heart's electrical activity.

asystole When no rhythm or electrical current is traveling through the cardiac conduction system.

atrial kick When blood is ejected into the ventricles by the atria immediately prior to ventricular systole.

atrioventricular (AV) node Specialized cells that delay the electrical conduction through the heart and allow the atria time to contract.

atrium (pl. atria) One of the upper two small chambers of the heart. The right atrium receives blood from the body through the vena cava, and the left atrium receives blood from the lungs through the pulmonary vein.

augmented Normally small ECG lead tracings that are increased in size by the ECG machine in order to be interpreted.

auscultation Listening to the body sounds, such as heart, lung, and stomach, using a stethoscope.

automatic external defibrillator (AED) A machine that analyzes the heart rhythm and will indicate the need for the heart to be shocked with energy to correct the irregular rhythm.

automaticity The ability of a cardiac cell to initiate an electrical impulse, without being stimulated by another source, causing a cardiac contraction.

B

beta blockers Drugs used to treat hypertension.

bigeminy Pattern in which every other complex is a premature beat.

biphasic The waveform that has an equally positive (upward) and negative (downward) deflection on the ECG tracing.

bipolar A type of ECG lead that measures the flow of electrical current in two directions at the same time.

blocked or nonconducted impulse Impulse occurs too soon after the preceding impulse, causing a period when no other impulses can occur in the ventricles.

bradycardia A slow heart rate, usually less than 60 beats per minute.

bundle branch block Impulse is delayed or blocked within the bundle branches of the normal conduction pathway.

bundle branches Left and right branches of the bundle of His that conduct impulses down either side of the interventricular septum to the left and right ventricles.

bundle of His (atrioventricular bundle) A bundle of fibers that originate in the AV node and enter the interventricular septum conducting electrical impulses to the left and right bundle branches.

C

capture The ability of the heart muscle to respond to electrical stimulation and depolarize the myocardial tissue.

cardiac cycle The period from the beginning of one heartbeat to the beginning of the next; the cardiac cycle is made up of the systole and diastole.

cardiac output parameters Observation guidelines used to assess the blood supply to the vital organs of the body to maintain normal function.

cardiologist A physician who specializes in the study of the heart.

cardiovascular Related to the heart and blood vessels (veins and arteries).

Code Blue The term is used by many institutions to describe when help is needed immediately for a person having a cardiac, respiratory, neurological condition. The patient is unresponsive, without a pulse or respirations. Other terms used to describe this situation may be *Dr. Blue, Dr. 999, Dr. Code*, and/or *MSET*. It is important to check your institution for its term used.

complexes Atrial or ventricular contractions as they appear on the ECG; complete ECG waveforms.

conductivity The ability of the heart cells to receive and transmit an electrical impulse.

congestive heart failure Failure of the heart to pump an adequate amount of blood to the body tissue.

contractility The ability of the heart muscle cells to shorten in response to an electrical stimulus.

coronary circulation The circulation of blood to and from the heart muscle.

coronary vascular disease (CVD) Narrowing of the arteries surrounding the heart causing a reduction in the blood flow to the heart.

D

defibrillator A machine that produces and sends an electrical shock to the heart, which is intended to correct the electrical pattern of the heart.

deoxygenated blood Blood that has little or minimal oxygen (oxygen-poor blood).

depolarization The electrical activation of the cells of the heart that initiates contraction of the heart muscle.

dextrocardia A congenital defect in which the major organs are reversed. The heart is located on the right side of the patient's chest.

diabetes mellitus (DM) A condition characterized by a lack of production of insulin resulting in elevated glucose (sugar) in the blood stream.

diastole The phase of the cardiac cycle when the heart is expanding and refilling; also known as the relaxation phase.

E

echocardiogram Noninvasive diagnostic test that uses sound to study the heart and blood vessels; also known as an ultrasound.

Einthoven triangle A triangle formed by three of the limb electrodes—the left arm, the right arm, and the left leg; it is used to determine the first six leads of the 12-lead ECG.

electrocardiogram (ECG) A tracing of the heart's electrical activity recorded by an electrocardiograph.

electrocardiograph An instrument used to record the electrical activity of the heart.

electrocardiology The study of the heart's electrical activity.

electrodes Small sensors, metal plates, or disposable units placed on the skin during an ECG to receive the electrical activity from the heart.

electronic pacemaker A device that delivers a small, measured amount of electrical energy to cause myocardial depolarization. Most artificial pacemakers are electronic.

excitability The ability of the heart muscle cells to respond to an impulse or stimulus.

F

false positive When a diagnostic test indicates that disease is present but in reality the test is negative and no disease is present.

focus or foci A cardiac cell or group of cells that function as an ectopic beat.

G

gain A control on the ECG machine that increases or decreases the size of the ECG tracing.

galvanometer An instrument that measures electrical current.

H

health care provider The scope of practice of each health care provider will determine the extent of the interpretation and treatment of each of the cardiac dysrhythmias or conditions. Each specific scope is determined by the licensure of each state. For example: Prescribing a medication is the responsibility of the physician. But some state practices allow nurse practitioners and physician assistants to prescribe medication under the guidance of the physician.

hepatitis Inflammation of the liver usually caused by a virus.

HIV (human immunodeficiency virus) The virus that causes AIDS (acquired immune deficiency syndrome).

Holter Proper name given to one type of ambulatory monitor, named after Norman Holter, inventor of the procedure and machine.

Holter monitor An instrument that records the electrical activity of the heart during a patient's normal daily activities; also known as an *ambulatory monitor*.

hypertension High blood pressure.

hyperventilate To breathe at an increased rate and depth of inspiration and expiration.

hypotension Condition in which the patient's blood pressure is not adequate to maintain good blood supply to the vital organs.

I

inhibited   Electrical current is stopped from being sent to the myocardium.

input   Data entered into an ECG machine, usually through electrodes on the skin surface.

intercostal space (ICS)   The space between two ribs.

interval   The period of time between two activities within the heart.

interventricular septum   A partition or wall (septum) that divides the right and left ventricles.

invasive   Procedure that requires entrance into a body cavity, tissue, or blood vessel.

ischemia   Lack of blood supply to an area of tissue due to a blockage in the circulation to that area.

isoelectric   The period when the electrical tracing of the ECG is at zero or a straight line, no positive or negative deflections are seen.

J

J point   A point on the QRS complex where the depolarization is completed and repolarization starts.

L

lead   A conductor attached to the ECG machine in the form of a covered wire.

left atrium   The left upper chamber of the heart, which receives blood from the lungs.

left ventricle   The left lower chamber of the heart, which pumps oxygenated blood through the body. It is the biggest and strongest chamber, known as the workhorse of the heart.

limb   An arm or a leg.

loss of capture   The pacing activity continues to occur without evidence that the electrical activity has depolarized or captured the myocardium.

M

malsensing   The pacemaker does not recognize or sense the patient's own inherent heartbeats.

midaxillary line   An imaginary vertical line that starts at the middle of the armpit.

midclavicular line   An imaginary line on the chest that runs vertically through the center of the clavicle.

midscapular line   Imaginary line on the back that runs vertically through the center of the scapula.

mitral (bicuspid) valve   Valve with two cusps or leaflets located between the left atrium and left ventricle; it prevents backflow of blood into the left atrium.

mm (millimeter)   A unit of measurement to indicate time on the ECG tracing. The time is measured on the horizontal axis.

multichannel recorder   An ECG machine that has the ability to record more than one lead tracing at a time, usually three, four, or six.

mV (millivolt)   A unit of measurement to indicate voltage on the ECG tracing. Voltage is measured on the vertical axis.

myocardial   Pertaining to the heart (*cardi*) muscle (*myo*).

myocardial infarction (MI) (heart attack)   A blockage of one or more of the coronary arteries causing lack of oxygen to the heart and damage to the muscle tissue.

N

neurological   Pertaining to the nervous system, its diseases, and its functions.

noninvasive   Procedure that does not require entrance into a body cavity, tissue, or blood vessel.

O

oscilloscope   A monitor or television-type device that shows the tracing of the electrical activity of the heart.

output display   The part of the ECG machine that displays the tracing for the electrical activity of the heart, usually in a printed form on a 12-lead ECG machine.

oversensing   The pacemaker senses electrical current from other muscle movements or electrical activity outside of the body as the patient's heart electrical current.

oxygenated blood   Blood having oxygen (oxygen-rich blood).

P

pacemaker   A cell or group of cells in the heart that affects the rate and rhythm of the heartbeat.

pacemaker (artificial)   A device that delivers a small, measured amount of electrical energy to cause myocardial depolarization. Most artificial pacemakers are electronic

pacemaker competition   Competition between the pacemaker generator and the heart's inherent rate over control of the myocardium.

pacemaker malfunctioning   The pacemaker fails to send an electrical impulse to the myocardium at the predetermined interval.

palpitations   Fast, irregular heartbeat sensation felt by the patient, which may or may not be associated with complaints of chest pain.

paraspinal line   Imaginary line on the spine that runs vertically through the side of the spine.

pericardium   A two-layered sac of tissue enclosing the heart.

polarization   The state of cellular rest in which the inside is negatively charged and the outside is positively charged.

posterior axillary line   Imaginary line on the back that runs vertically from the shoulder down on the outer edge of the rib cage.

precordial   A type of lead placed on the chest in front of the heart; known as a V lead.

pulmonary artery   Large artery that transports deoxygenated blood from the right ventricle to the lungs. This is the only artery in the body that carries deoxygenated blood.

pulmonary circulation   The transportation of blood to and from the lungs; blood is oxygenated in the lungs during pulmonary circulation.

pulmonary semilunar valve   A valve found in the pulmonary artery that prevents backflow of blood into the right ventricle during pulmonary circulation.

pulmonary vein   A blood vessel that transports blood from the lungs to the left atrium. The only vein in the body to carry oxygenated blood.

Purkinje fibers   The fibers within the heart that distribute electrical impulses from cell to cell throughout the ventricles.

Purkinje network   A network of fibers that distribute electrical impulses through the ventricles; named after a scientist with the last name of Purkinje.

Q

quadgeminy   Pattern in which every fourth complex is a premature beat.

R

repolarization   When heart muscle cells return to their resting electrical state and the heart muscle relaxes.

rhythm   The regularity of an occurrence such as the heartbeat.

right atrium   The right upper chamber of the heart, which receives blood from the body.

right ventricle   The right lower chamber of the heart, which pumps blood to the lungs.

S

segment   A portion or part of the electrical tracing produced by the heart.

seizure   An interruption of the electrical activity in the brain that causes involuntary muscle movement and sometimes unconsciousness.

semilunar valve   A valve with half-moon-shaped cusps that open and close, allowing blood to travel only one way; located in the pulmonary artery and the aorta.

signal processing   The process within the ECG machine that amplifies the electrical impulse and converts it to a mechanical action on the output display.

single-channel recorder   An ECG machine that records one lead tracing at a time.

sinoatrial (SA) node   An area of specialized cells in the upper right atrium that initiates the heartbeat.

skin rasp   A rough piece of material used to abrade (scrape) the skin prior to electrode placement.

somatic tremor   Voluntary or involuntary muscle movement; also known as body tremor.

speed   A control on the ECG machine that regulates how fast or slow the paper runs during the tracing.

standardization   Setting of the ECG machine output so that 1 millivolt equals 1 centimeter.

stat   Immediately.

stress ECG   Another name for exercise electrocardiography.

stylus   A pointed, penlike instrument that uses heat to record electrical impulses on the ECG graph paper.

suprasternal notch   The dip you feel at the base of the neck just above where the clavicle attaches to the sternum.

supraventricular   An ectopic focus originating above the ventricles in the atria or junctional region of the heart.

syncope   Condition when the patient loses consciousness (fainting).

systemic circulation   The circulation between the heart and the entire body, excluding the lungs.

systole   The contraction phase of the cardiac cycle, during which the heart is pumping blood out to the body.

T

tachycardia   A fast heart rate, usually greater than 100 beats per minute.

target heart rate (THR)   Heart rate measurement needed to truly exercise the heart; determined by 220 minus the patient's age.

technician   An individual who has the knowledge and skills to carry out technical procedures.

technologist   An individual who specializes in a field of science.

telemetry   The transmission of data electronically to an unattached or distant location.

thallium stress test   An invasive type of exercise electrocardiography in which thallium, a radiopaque substance (one that is visible with an x-ray machine), is injected into the body to permit viewing the vessels around the heart.

tricuspid valve   Valve located between the right atrium and right ventricle; it prevents backflow of blood into the right atrium.

trigeminy   Pattern in which every third complex is a premature beat.

triggered   Electrical current is sent from the pacemaker generator to the myocardium to cause the depolarization of the myocardial tissue.

U

unipolar   A type of ECG lead that measures the flow of electrical current in one direction only.

V

vagal tone   Condition in which impulses over the vagus nerve exert a continuous inhibitory effect upon the heart and cause a decrease in heart rate.

vena cava   Largest vein in the body, which provides a pathway for deoxygenated blood to return to the heart; its upper portion, the superior vena cava, transports blood from the head, arms, and upper body; and its lower portion, the inferior vena cava, transports blood from the lower body and legs.

W

wandering baseline   When the tracing of an ECG drifts away from the center of the paper; also called baseline shift. It has many causes, which can be corrected.

Credits

Index

Page references followed by *f* or *t* indicate entries in figures or tables, respectively.

Atrioventricular (AV) block
  first degree, 140–141, 140*f*
  second degree, Mobitz type I, 141–142, 142*f*,
    144, 144*t*
  second degree, Mobitz type II, 143–144, 143*f*, 144*t*
  third degree, 143, 144–146, 145*f*
Atrioventricular (AV) bundle, 38, 39*f*, 39*t*
Atrioventricular (AV) delay, with electronic
    pacemakers, 159–160, 161
Atrioventricular (AV) node, 38, 39*f*, 39*t*
  rhythms originating from, 135–137
Atrioventricular pacemakers, 158–160, 159*f*
Atrioventricular valves, 30, 30*t*, 31*f*
Atrium (pl. atria), 29–31, 31*f*, 32*f*
  circulatory role of, 33–34, 34*f*
  rhythms originating from, 128–135
Augmented leads, 55–56, 57*f*
Automatic external defibrillators (AEDs),
    10–12, 11*f*
Automaticity, 36–38, 132, 135
Autonomic nervous system (ANS), 37
AV. *See* Atrioventricular
aVF lead, 56, 57*f*
aVL lead, 56, 57*f*
aVR lead, 56, 57*f*

B

Baseline ECG, 6, 8
Baseline shift, 92, 93*f*, 93*t*, 94–95, 94*f*
  causes of, 93*t*, 94–95
  correction of, 93*t*, 95
Beta blockers, and exercise ECG, 190–191
Bicuspid (mitral) valve, 30–31, 30*t*, 31*f*, 32*f*, 33
  opening and closing of, 35, 36*f*
Bicuspid valve regurgitation, acute, 132
Bigeminy, 149*t*
Billing, 98
Bipolar leads, 55
Blocked impulses, 141
Blood pressure
  abnormal, reporting of, 186
  elevated (hypertension), 2, 193
  in exercise testing, 185–186, 187, 194–198
  healthy, maintenance of, 2*t*
Blood vessels, 31–32, 32*f*. *See also* Circulation
Body tremor, 92, 93–94, 93*f*, 93*t*
  causes of, 93–94, 93*t*
  correction of, 93*t*, 94
Bradycardia, 63, 117
  sinus, 122, 123–124, 124*f*
Breast(s), and lead placement, 86–87, 102
Breast implants, 102
Bruce protocol, for exercise ECG, 196*t*
Bundle branch(es), 38, 39*f*, 39*t*, 122

Bundle branch block, 146, 147*f*
Bundle branch block dysrhythmias, 146–148
Bundle of His, 38, 39*f*, 39*t*, 122

C

Calcium, 38
Calibration, of ECG machine, 64–65, 65*f*, 69
Calipers, 115, 116*f*
Capture, 159–161
  loss of, 161, 162*t*
Cardiac arrest, 157
  emergency measures in, 10–12, 105
  sinus, 127–128, 127*f*, 129
Cardiac care unit (CCU), 7
Cardiac conduction system, 36–39, 39*f*, 39*t*
Cardiac control center, 37–38
Cardiac cycle, 35–36
Cardiac medications, 81, 209, 218
Cardiac output, decreased
  with accelerated idioventricular rhythm, 152
  with agonal rhythm, 155
  with atrial fibrillation, 134
  with atrial flutter, 133
  with idioventricular rhythm, 151
  with junctional rhythm, 137
  with premature atrial complexes, 130
  with premature junctional complex, 136
  with premature ventricular complexes, 150
  with second degree atrioventricular block, Mobitz
    type I, 142
  with second degree atrioventricular block, Mobitz
    type II, 143
  signs and symptoms of, 123, 123*t*
  with sinus arrest, 128
  with sinus bradycardia, 124
  with sinus tachycardia, 125
  with supraventricular dysrhythmia, 139
  with third degree atrioventricular block, 145–146
  with ventricular tachycardia, 153
Cardiac output, normal, 123
Cardiac output parameters, 141
Cardiac veins, 34*f*
Cardiologist, 188
Cardiopulmonary resuscitation (CPR), 12, 194
Cardiovascular disease, 2
Cardiovascular system, 27–43
Care of equipment, 17*t*, 99–100, 100*f*, 101*f*
Cassette-recorder ambulatory monitor, 224
CCU (cardiac/coronary care unit), 7
Centers for Disease Control and Prevention (CDC),
    14–15
Cerebral vascular accident (CVA), 134
Chambers of heart, 29–31, 31*f*
CHB (complete heart block), 143, 144–146, 145*f*

ECG machine—*Cont.*
  operation of, 91–92
  output display of, 60–61
  signal processing in, 60
  single-channel, 59–60, 60*f*, 81, 98, 99*f*
  size and weight of, 59
  speed of, 62
  standardization of, 64–65, 65*f*, 69, 92
  storage in, 61
  stylus of, 64
  types of, 59–60
Echocardiogram, 198
Education, patient, 16–18
  on ambulatory monitoring, 216–219, 219*t*
  on exercise electrocardiography, 188–192
e-ICU, 8
18-lead ECG, 103–105
Einthoven, Wilhelm, 4, 40
Einthoven triangle, 55, 55*f*, 56*f*, 57*f*
Elderly patients, 103, 222
Electrical impulses of conduction, 36–39
Electrical stimulation and ECG waveform, 40
Electricity and ECG, 4
Electrocardiogram, 2
Electrocardiograph (ECG), 2, 3*f. See also specific*
    entries
  AHA recommendation on, 6
  baseline, 6, 8
  components of, 40–42, 41*t*, 42*f*
  conditions evaluated by, 8, 9*t*
  in doctors' offices or ambulatory care clinics, 8–10
  documentation of, 20, 20*t*
  electrical stimulation and, 40
  electricity and, 4
  equipment for, 2, 3*f*, 14, 17*t*, 53–72
  exercise, 8–9, 9*f*, 183–199
  functions of, 60–62
  history of, 4
  in hospital (acute care), 7
  interpretation of, 4, 61, 113–163
  normal tracing in, 6, 7*f*
  outside health care facility, 10–13
  pediatric, 101, 102*f*
  performance of, 2–3
  preparation for, 80–81, 91, 101
  reasons for performing, 3
  serial, 66–67, 94
  special patient considerations in, 102–105
  uses of, 6–7
Electrocardiographer, role of, 5
Electrocardiology, 4
Electrodes, 53, 55, 60, 66–67
  alligator-type clips for, 87, 100, 100*f*
  for ambulatory monitoring, 222–223, 222*f*, 223*f*
  application or placement of, 85–88
  cleaning and maintenance of, 100

Electrodes—*Cont.*
  definition of, 66
  disposable, 66–67, 66*f*, 100
  for exercise ECG, 194, 195*f*
  handling and storage of, 67
  mixing of, inaccuracy with, 66
  for pediatric patients, 101, 102*f*
  relocation of, 89
  reusable, 66, 100
  silver, 66–67
Electronic pacemaker(s), 5, 157–162
  ambulatory monitoring of, 209–210, 212–213
  atrial, 158–159, 159*f*
  atrioventricular, 158–160, 159*f*
  atrioventricular delay with, 159–160, 161
  for bundle branch block, 148
  capture with, 159–161
  chamber depolarization characteristics of, 159
  complications of, 161–162, 162*t*
  definition of, 157
  evaluating function of, 159–160
  evaluating tracing with, 160–161
  implantation of, 157, 158*f*
  loss of capture with, 161, 162*t*
  malfunctioning, 161, 162*t*
  malsensing, 161, 162*t*
  oversensing, 161, 162*t*
  pacing spike of, 159, 159*f*
  safety of, 158
  for third degree atrioventricular block, 146
  25 percent intervals of, 160
  ventricular, 158–159, 159*f*
Embolism, 134
Emergencies, 7, 10–12, 105
  asystole, 157
  bundle branch block, 148
  communication in, 157
  crash cart for, 156
  exercise ECG, 192–193, 193*t*
  second degree atrioventricular block, Mobitz type
    II, 143
  third degree atrioventricular block, 146
  ventricular fibrillation, 156
  ventricular tachycardia, 154
Emergency room (ER), 7
Emphysema, 132
Endocardium, 29, 29*t*, 30*f*
Environmental control, 17*t*
Epicardium, 28–29, 29*t*, 30*f*
Equipment, 2, 3*f*, 14, 17*t*, 53–72. *See also specific types*
  for ambulatory monitoring, 221, 221*f*
  for exercise ECG, 184*f*, 193–194
  maintenance of, 99–100, 100*f*, 101*f*
  for pediatric patients, 101, 102*f*
Escape beats, 153
Ethics, 19

R

Rate pressure product (RPP), 198
RBBB (right bundle branch block), 146–147, 147*f*
Records, 20, 20*t*, 83
   maintenance of, 69
Refusal by patient, 83, 190, 191*t*
Regularity, 115–116
Regular rhythm, heart rate calculation in, 116–117, 119*t*
Relaxation of heart, 35, 36*f*
Renal infarction, 134
Repolarization, 40–42
Reporting results, 97–98, 123
   of ambulatory monitoring, 224–225
Requisition, 80–81
Respiratory arrest, 105
Results, reporting of, 97–98, 123, 224–225
Reusable electrodes, 66, 100
Rhythm(s). *See also specific rhythms*
   determination of, 115–116, 116*f*
   heart block, 140–146
   identifying components of, 115–121
   irregular, heart rate calculation in, 117–118
   normal sinus, 119*t*, 122–123, 122*f*
   originating from atria, 128–135
   originating from atrioventricular node, 135–137
   originating from sinoatrial node, 122–128
   originating from ventricles, 149–157
   regular, heart rate calculation in, 116–117, 119*t*
Rhythm strip, 102, 115–121
Ribs, as anatomical landmark, 84
Right atrium, 29–30, 31*f*, 32*f*
   circulatory role of, 33–34, 34*f*
Right bundle branch, 38, 39*f*
Right bundle branch block (RBBB), 146–147, 147*f*
Right coronary artery, 33–34, 34*f*
Right marginal artery, 34*f*
Right pulmonary artery, 31*f*, 32*f*
Right pulmonary veins, 31*f*
Right ventricle, 29–30, 31*f*, 32*f*
   circulatory role of, 33, 34*f*
R-on-T PVCs, 149*t*, 150
Room conditions, 80
Routine ECG, in hospital setting, 7
RPP (rate pressure product), 198
R-R interval, 42
   in accelerated idioventricular rhythm, 152
   in agonal rhythm, 154
   in asystole, 156
   in atrial fibrillation, 133
   in atrial flutter, 132
   calculating heart rate from, 69–70, 70*f*, 70*t*, 116–117, 119*t*
   in first degree atrioventricular block, 141
   in idioventricular rhythm, 151

R-R interval—*Cont.*
   in junctional rhythm, 137
   measurement of, 116, 118*f*
   in premature atrial complexes, 129
   in premature ventricular complexes, 150
   in second degree atrioventricular block, Mobitz type I, 142
   in second degree atrioventricular block, Mobitz type II, 143
   in sinus arrest, 127
   in sinus bradycardia, 124
   in sinus dysrhythmia, 126
   in sinus tachycardia, 125
   in supraventricular tachycardia, 138
   in third degree atrioventricular block, 145
   in ventricular fibrillation, 155
   in ventricular tachycardia, 152
R wave, 40, 42
   measurement of, 118
   in sinus rhythm, 122

S

Safety, 89–92, 90*t*
   crash cart, 156
   electricity and ECG, 4
   electronic pacemaker, 158
   exercise ECG, 186, 192–193, 194, 196
   guidelines for, 14
   handling ambulatory monitors, 211
   mixing of electrodes, 66
SA node. *See* Sinoatrial node
Scanner, 10
Scope of practice, 139, 218
Second degree atrioventricular block
   Mobitz type I, 141–142, 142*f*, 144, 144*t*
   Mobitz type II, 143–144, 143*f*, 144*t*
Segments, ECG, 40–42. *See also specific types*
Seizures, 105
Self-adhesive electrodes, 66
Semilunar valves, 30, 30*t*, 31*f*, 32*f*, 33, 34*f*
Serial ECGs, 66–67, 94
Shockable rhythm, 11
SICU (surgical intensive care unit), 7
Signal processing, 60
Silver electrodes, 66–67
Single-channel recorder, 59–60, 60*f*
   paper for, 81
   tracings of, 59–60, 98, 99*f*
Sinoatrial (SA) node, 38, 39*f*, 39*t*, 122
   rhythms originated from, 122–128
Sinus arrest, 127–128, 127*f*, 129
Sinus bradycardia, 122, 123–124, 124*f*
Sinus dysrhythmia, 122, 126–127, 126*f*
Sinus rhythm, normal, 119*t*, 122–123, 122*f*